THE
OWL DIET

D1319591

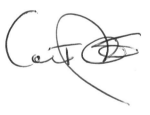

Carter O. Abbott, M.D.

ISBN: 978-1-57579-435-8

Library of Congress Control Number: 2010943030

Printed in the United States of America

PINE HILL PRESS
4000 West 57th Street
Sioux Falls, SD 57106

Thanks go to my

loyal bearded companions,
past and present,

Brimley, Gryphon and Cayenne
for their unconditional love and affection

Acknowledgements

Thank you to the following people who made this happen:

- To Dr. Simeons who first reported the use of HCG with a very low calorie diet.

- To the first thousand people who undertook the OWL Diet with me – their experiences formed the backbone of this book. By observation and keen listening, I learned with them what works, and what does not.

- To my wife Lenore who has followed me on a long career in medicine and has always offered unconditional support and love for all my ideas and dreams.

- To Tom Kerr who visually captured the OWL Diet and provided the great illustrations for this book.

- To Matthew Samp who opened doors to the world of writing and publishing for my first book.

Table of Contents

Introduction

PART IV: GETTING AND STAYING ON TRACK

About the Author

Introduction

As a medical doctor, I have treated thousands of obese patients. I was good at writing prescriptions for their high blood pressure, heart disease and diabetes. But I was not good at getting them to lose weight. I treated their diseases, but not the underlying problem: their obesity.

Furthermore, I was unable to treat my own obesity problem with the standard advice to eat less and exercise more. That was before I learned about HCG and low calorie dieting. I used HCG to lose weight quickly, safely and permanently. So did my wife.

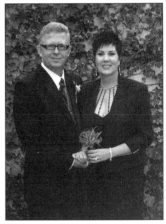

Before the OWL Diet.

Through those experiences, I developed a low calorie diet (LCD) that works! I call it the OWL (Omaha Weight Loss) Diet. I have updated the original HCG Diet as described by Dr. A.T.W. Simeons decades ago. The OWL Diet provides for more calories and food variety. The result is a realistic diet that results in fast and successful weight loss. And just as important, you learn how to keep the weight off permanently.

Learn the OWL Diet. Focus and commit, follow it completely and you will be surprised how easy it is to lose weight. The OWL Diet can be fun, exciting and empowering. Weight loss is a journey, not a race, but the OWL Diet will reward you every week for your short-term sacrifices.

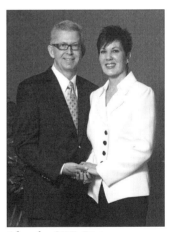

After the OWL Diet.

Carter Abbott, M.D.
Omaha, Nebraska, USA
January 2011

PART I:

THE BASICS

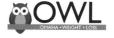

Chapter 1
THE ROAD TO PERMANENT WEIGHT LOSS

Perhaps you're like so many of my patients who struggle their entire lives with excess weight. Maybe you've tried every diet under the sun without success, or worse yet, you've lost the excess weight only to put it back on and more.

You know the humiliation of trying to squeeze into one of those tiny airline seats or of caving in to the cravings for a piece of pizza or an ice cream cone and note the accusing stares of those around you. You know the pain of joints forced to support more weight than their designer intended and perhaps the very real threat of an early death from heart disease or stroke and certain types of cancer associated with obesity.

Doctors like myself have probably (sometimes rather sanctimoniously) proclaimed that you simply need to "eat less and exercise more."

You know you're not alone. Whether your spare tire is 20 pounds, like mine was, or you have a dangerous 100 pounds or more to lose, I have found a way to make that happen.

I know this may sound like one of those late night infomercials, but bear with me. I know the plan I have developed called the OWL Diet (Omaha Weight Loss Diet) actually works. It worked for me and it's worked for hundreds of my patients who have lost their excess weight and kept it off.

My story may be a lot like yours:

As I got into my late 30s, my weight started to inch upwards. In just a few years, I had a stubborn 20 pound "spare tire" that simply would not go away. For more than a decade, I struggled with that "spare tire."

I really got serious about it in 1998 when I decided to take the advice I had given to hundreds of patients over my 25 years of medical practice.

As a medical doctor, I thought I knew the answer: Take in fewer calories and exercise more. Oh sure, I could lose a few pounds. I could sweat and exercise until I was blue in the face, but I couldn't get rid of those last few pounds.

After six months of working the treadmill, stretching, lifting weights and sweating, I was successful in losing 14 pounds. My progress then came to a roaring halt when one day, during a bench press, I experienced a sudden pain in my neck and numbness down my right arm. I was unable to lift more than 10 pounds, run or bend my neck without experiencing a surge of pain. Without the exercise, all of my weight "returned" and then some.

The neck and arm pain continued and eventually I chose to undergo neck surgery that would forever limit running or heavy lifting, which might cause further neck problems.

Then in 2004, I tore the medial meniscus (cartilage) in my right knee while I was working in the yard.

The end result of my two injuries was that my weight shot up to 209 pounds, a 25-pound weight gain.

With obesity, my health had suffered. I developed hypertension (high blood pressure), I snored at night and my knees and back ached. At 5'10", I was overweight and I knew it, but I could not get past the "complaining stage."

I was still able to enjoy day hiking with my wife, Lenore. During hiking trips to the mountains we were very active, walking up to eight miles a day and no doubt burning many calories. What I noticed was that associated with all of the healthy physical activity was a very brisk, if not ravenous, appetite. We were hungry and responded to the urge by eating more granola, fruit, breads and meats. At the end of each hiking trip we felt renewed and refreshed, but we also never lost any weight!

It seemed like there was nothing I could do to rid myself of the extra weight.

Then I began to notice a common thread among some of my patients who were taking Human Chorionic Gonadotropin (HCG), a hormone naturally produced by pregnant women. HCG has profound effects on metabolism during pregnancy. In the non-pregnant state, it appears to suppress appetite and helps to mobilize fat out of the body.

Typically, these patients on the HCG Diet were losing three to five pounds a week while keeping their energy levels high and their hunger in check.

Intrigued and more than a little excited, I decided to make myself a human guinea pig for this concept. Despite her initial hesitation, Lenore my wife and life partner joined me on this journey of weight loss over the next five weeks.

Both of us were surprised by how well we felt. Although there were times of hunger, we stayed committed and were greatly encouraged when we saw the pounds melt away.

To make a long story short, I lost 20 pounds and Lenore lost 16 pounds in five weeks using HCG injections and a Low Calorie Diet (LCD). The meat, vegetables and fruit helped us lose weight rapidly. The HCG OWL Diet also taught us how to make healthier eating a permanent part of our lifestyle.

Well, you might say, a low calorie diet will make anyone lose weight, but who wants to be miserably hungry?

First, we weren't miserable at all. Like most people on the OWL Diet, we had occasional hunger pangs, but it wasn't anything we couldn't cope with. Some people have complete hunger control, but it is important to note that for success on the OWL Diet, you must have a total commitment to your weight loss goal. For most of us, HCG helps curb hunger and cravings, but it is not a magic bullet.

And, secondly, we didn't gain our weight back when we stopped taking the HCG injections. Two years later, I effortlessly maintain my weight at 182 pounds on my 5'10"-inch frame. The BMI chart says I am still overweight and it is my goal to get to my ideal weight of 175 pounds - right in the healthy weight zone.

As a medical doctor, I have cared for thousands of people with diabetes mellitus, heart disease, hypertension and arthritis over the years. Many of these patients were also obese.

My efforts to help them lose weight with the traditional dictum of "eat less and exercise more" was not getting them anywhere.

My personal experience with low calorie dieting and HCG convinced me I could offer patients at my medical spa here in Omaha some real hope with a safe and effective program of medical grade weight loss. I know it works because I've experienced it for myself.

As a physician, I had safety and effectiveness in mind when I developed the Omaha Weight Loss (OWL) Diet. I was not comfortable with the older version of Very Low Calorie Dieting (VLCD) of 500 calories per day as described by Dr. A.T. W. Simeons more than 70 years ago. I have introduced the safety of a higher calorie allowance while ensuring weight loss success. The term Low Calorie Diet (LCD) has been developed to describe my allowed range of food and beverage choices that results in an average intake of 600-700 calories per day with the OWL Diet.

I also believe that the original HCG Diet added unnecessary rules and myths that can now be discarded. I do not complicate the message with reference to phases, but rather distinguish between fat loading, low calorie dieting and making healthier long-term maintenance food choices.

This book gives you the tools for success. When you are ready to experience life long weight loss, then apply these principles, and achieve your own weight loss success story. Weight loss takes commitment and focus, skills that when applied to other challenges in life will also lead to other positive results.

We have guided hundreds of individuals to permanent weight loss at our medical spa. With this book, I hope that thousands more may benefit.

The OWL Diet is not to be undertaken without proper medical supervision. HCG is a prescription medication that can only be obtained in the United States with a valid doctor's prescription. I see all of my OWL Diet patients weekly.

A QUICK LOOK AT THE OWL DIET

Here it is, the OWL Diet in brief summary:

- **Meat:** 7 oz. of very lean chicken, fish, shrimp, scallops, beef or game meat daily. You'll be weighing all your meat on a food scale before it is cooked.

- **Vegetables:** 4 cups prepared any way you like, without any fat.
- **Salad greens and celery:** unlimited quantities.
- **Grain carbohydrates:** up to 120 calories a day, such as a whole grain sandwich round, Wasa cracker or Melba toast.
- **Fruit:** 2 servings of fruit daily.
- **Water:** drink at least 68 oz. (2 liters) daily.
- **Beverages:** include coffee, tea and other zero-calorie drinks. Caffeine, artificial sweeteners and sugar-free sodas are permitted.
- **Alcohol:** You may also have 1 alcoholic beverage daily if you wish.
- **You'll be using HCG shots** or transdermal cream daily. (Don't worry, it's a small needle and you'll quickly become very comfortable with administering your own intramuscular injections).

You do not have to count the calories of your food, although some people choose to do so. By selecting a variety of foods from the lists of approved foods, you will average 600-700 calories per day, and lose an average of 15-20 pounds per month.

In future chapters, I'll be going into much more detail about the OWL Diet, the changes I have made compared to the original HCG Diet and my reasons for them.

It is with great satisfaction that I have finally found a way to safely and effectively help patients lose weight and live a healthier life! Weight loss not only works as primary prevention to avoid developing certain health problems, but also to treat and even eradicate certain medical conditions.

My personal experience continues to serve me and my patients.

I have been able to stop my medication for high blood pressure. My acid reflux is greatly reduced and I now rarely require the use of acid suppression medication. My back and knee pain are greatly improved. Irritable bowel symptoms are now rarely encountered as my wife and I continue to make healthier food choices. Many of my patients have experienced the same improvement in their health.

We have both been successful in maintaining a healthy weight. Weight loss for us has been a "one-way journey." I encourage all of our weight loss clients to share the same goal. Lenore and I are not going back to being overweight. Both of us took great pleasure from giving our "fat clothes" away and buying new ones!

Losing weight has been a boost to our self-esteem and we have discovered a renewed commitment to healthier living. Weight control is a permanent fixture in our lives. I tell our patients that with the Omaha Weight Loss (OWL)

Diet they'll learn how to lose weight and during their personal weight loss journey they'll also learn how to keep it off for life!

One of the greatest surprises of the OWL Diet for Lenore and me was learning that we could consume fewer calories and yet feel well, with adequate levels of energy and excellent clarity of thought. Before OWL, we thought we had a fairly healthy diet, with plentiful use of fresh fruits and vegetables. Like many others, we did not realize that our portion sizes were out of control.

We also overindulged in foods that have now become special treats, such as desserts, sweets, cookies and ice cream. My wife and I are now able to enjoy all of the foods that we had in the past, but with a new knowledge regarding portion control and the need to make treats a special event, not a daily event. We also learned that we were consuming excessive carbohydrates in the form of breads. We now enjoy bread, but in very limited quantities.

Likewise, our use of fats and oils was also excessive. Before the OWL Diet, my wife always had half and half cream on hand for her coffee - one quart at work and one at home. I never thought that I would see the day when she would drink black coffee, but it happened! We have always used healthy oil to cook with, but have learned that smaller amounts of oil are more than adequate.

SETTING YOUR WEIGHT LOSS GOAL

The first step is to calculate your Body Mass Index, or BMI for short. The United States government has established the BMI as a standard for physicians to follow. The easiest way to find your own BMI is to go to a web page posted by the National Institute of Health at: www.nhlbisupport.com/bmi

Simply enter your current height and weight and the web calculator will tell you your BMI.

If your BMI is 25-29.9 then you are considered to be overweight.

If your BMI is 30-39.9 then you fall within the range of obesity.

If your BMI is 40 or higher, then you are considered to be morbidly obese.

You may find a healthy weight goal appears too low. I suggest that you set a first weight loss goal that is achievable within the first four to eight weeks. Losing weight is a journey, not a race! It is important to feel a sense of accomplishment for each increment of weight that is lost.

BMI calculations are only a guide. I have found that if you are under 5'3" or over 6'0", modifications are often needed based on body build and the amount of muscle mass that is present.

Typically you will lose the most weight during your first week on the OWL Diet. A common mistake is to then set the bar too high for subsequent weeks. Look at your overall weight loss progress over an entire month. Avoid weighing yourself at home every day. Instead, weigh in weekly with your doctor who is supervising the OWL Diet.

Remember that men, young people, tall people and people who have the most weight to lose often lose weight faster.

The average weight loss seen per month is 15 pounds for women 20 pounds for men. If you are a 70 year old female at 5'0", then losing at a rate of 8-10 pounds a month would be an excellent result.

As you get closer to your weight loss goal, your rate of weight loss may also slow.

You may take a break during your weight loss journey. This may be mandated by illness or the need to have surgery. Breaks are also often taken during business trips and personal vacations. Your doctor will work with you to help you choose the correct food selection and calorie intake during your break.

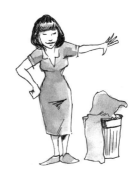

Chapter 2
THE OWL DIET
KEYS TO SUCCESS

By participating in the OWL Diet, you will learn that reducing calories is the secret to successful rapid weight loss. When you consume a Low Calorie Diet (LCD), your body is driven to burn fat stores for sources of additional energy. If your body needs a total of 2,500 calories per day, and you limit your intake to 700 calories, then your body is driven to look for the difference - and burns fat to generate the additional 1,800 calories. This is the secret to losing three to five pounds per week.

THE "WOW" FACTOR

There's not doubt about it: When you get on the scale after your first week on the OWL Diet and you see your weight has dropped by four to ten pounds, you get a rush of satisfaction.

The success of a weight loss program is as much psychological as it is physical. I found I was actually eager to get on the scale each week to find another three to five pounds gone and the same amount every week thereafter.

Conventional weight control programs promise a weight loss of a pound or two a week. While these small losses are admirable, they aren't very exciting. If you have 100 pounds to lose and you start doing the math, you realize you'll be slogging along at the pace of a pound or so a week for two years. Quite honestly, it's depressing and you're likely to give up shortly after you start.

If you're reading this book, you've no doubt already done the math in your head. Let's say you have 50 pounds to lose. You could lose it in as little as ten weeks—just two and a half months. At worst, as long as you are truly faithful to the diet, it could take you just over four months. That seems achievable to almost anyone.

I can't emphasize enough that you'll be making permanent changes to your eating habits, but the maintenance diet is nowhere near as stringent as the weight loss plan. After your weight loss on the OWL Diet, you'll feel so good that you will want to continue on with a healthy eating program.

I know that hunger is a huge issue with dieting. Nobody enjoys the sensation of being hungry. With HCG, and other medication if necessary, your hunger will be reduced and manageable. Hunger control will give you the willpower to forge ahead to your goal.

LIMITED EXERCISE

You will be limiting your exercise while you are on the OWL Diet.

In fact, I've seen patients who did not heed my advice on exercise, and continued to participate in high-energy fitness activities (such as "Boot Camps," spinning classes and jogging). They did very poorly.

Without exception, this group struggles with hunger and "exercisers" are forced to increase their intake of calories beyond that allowed with the LCD. The result is what I call "cheating" or eating more than the LCD allows. Weight loss is slowed and patients feel both discouraged and guilty.

After two to three weeks of high levels of exercise, many of these participants wisely revert to lower levels of activity, with the result that they have better energy, can follow the OWL Diet exactly, and lose three to five pounds per week.

Please understand that I want you to have an active lifestyle that includes regular exercise. Exercise is vital for physical and emotional well-being. Exercise helps control blood pressure, regulate blood sugar, and strengthen the heart and lungs. Joints maintain mobility, muscles remain toned and balance is maintained with regular exercise. As we age, mobility is intimately connected to independent living and quality of life.

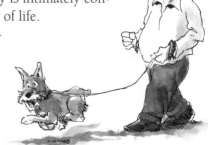

On the OWL Diet, you'll be encouraged to get 20-30 minutes of mild exercise every day: easy walking, slow bicycle riding or yoga. For exercise haters, this is another boost to help you be successful on the OWL Diet.

Medical studies are now showing that once you achieve your weight loss goal, then regular exercise is very important to maintaining your healthy weight. Once you attain your weight loss goal, you are strongly encouraged to have an active lifestyle that includes regular exercise.

The Key to Controlling Hunger is to Limit your Amount of Exercise.

When my wife and I go for lengthy bicycle rides or hiking in the mountains, we are exerting a lot of energy and are burning off a lot of calories. We also notice that we are constantly eating. The increased level of physical activity drives us to have increased hunger. I have always enjoyed hiking trips, but have never lost weight during any of them.

For years, my patients have told me how hard they "worked out" with exercise and how disappointed they were with the rate of weight loss. The reality is that science is now showing that exercise is a slow way to lose weight. Once again, the message about exercise has to be clearly stated: It's good for you, but it's not a fast way to lose weight.

I have met many men and women who thought they ate a healthy diet and exercised regularly, but could not achieve their ideal body weight. They complained about stubborn regional fat deposits in the abdomen, back and thigh areas that they were unable to lose with conventional dieting and exercise. By following the OWL Diet, these individuals were able to mobilize fat and burn off unwanted fat deposits. Once an ideal weight and shape is accomplished, they are able to return to a very active exercise regimen. These individuals are using the OWL Diet with a goal of body sculpting. The OWL Diet helps them achieve the appearance that they desire, without the risks associated with surgical procedures like liposuction.

The Key to a Healthy Diet is to Eat Healthy Food.

It may seem obvious that healthy food makes for a successful diet, but in fact many diets require excessive amounts of certain food groups (such as proteins) or total avoidance of others (such as grain carbohydrates). They do not always offer enough of a healthy balance of the food groups.

Other diet programs have you drink prepared shakes. These shakes have calories, but they are not real food. Finally there are the very commercialized programs that have you buy their prepared and manufactured foods.

Some of these foods may even resemble foods that you really should not be eating (such as pizzas or brownies), but a method has been found to lower the fat calories of those foods, so that you can still lose weight.

My concern with shakes and prepared foods is what you'll eat once you have lost your weight. I now know that to be an effective long term program of weight control, there needs to be a permanent change in food behavior. Food behavior includes shopping for groceries, cooking food properly at home and learning to say "No" to frequent excesses of breads, oils, desserts and other treats.

With the OWL Diet, you are eating fresh or frozen fresh foods. These are real foods grown and raised on the earth. You will be eating healthy lean meats as well as healthy amounts of fresh fruits and vegetables. These are the foods that our bodies were designed to eat! It is no wonder that so many people on the OWL Diet feel healthier, have excellent energy, better cognitive function, improved sleep and relief of irritable bowel problems. Some participants feel like they are "detoxifying" as they learn to avoid processed and manufactured foods that have less nutritional value and are often full of chemical additives.

Over a period of weeks to months on the OWL Diet, you will learn what you were doing wrong in the past. Your food behavior change will be your secret to the maintenance of your weight loss.

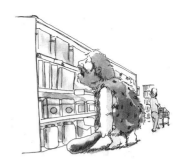

Chapter 3
WHY WE OVEREAT

THE "FRUITS OF OUR LABOR"

We no longer eat to survive. We eat out of habit. We eat of out boredom. We eat for comfort. We eat because we are worried or stressed or unhappy. We eat because we are addicted to sugar and salt. We eat because there is a tempting array of foods and so-called foods available to us that are fast, affordable and readily available. On that list are junk foods and highly processed foods that are laden with salt, high fructose corn syrup and preservatives that transform them from anything remotely resembling food to something that can actually be harmful to your health.

Our ancestors would have been flabbergasted by the variety of foods available in the average American supermarket. For most of human existence, humans needed to hunt and gather wild foods to survive. It was a full-time job for both man and woman to hunt for game and gather edible plants, roots, seeds, nuts and berries not only to survive in the warm season, but also to survive the long cold winters. Not only was it time consuming, the act of feeding an individual or a family was also physically demanding, whether it involved tracking herds for dozens of miles or trekking through forests and plains to find edible plant material. Only those who were able to provide for themselves survived; ensuring a strengthening human race of resourceful and capable hunters and gatherers. Hunters and gatherers certainly were not prone to obesity!

As society advanced, a regular supply of food was a benchmark for success and strength. The survival of monarchs and governments could hinge on the reliability of food supplies for their people, so governments encouraged agriculture for their own political purposes and to create a more stable society.

Unlike the days when our ancestors spent days tracking animals, searching for edible plants or toiling in their fields, we modern humans can get an absurd abundance of food simply by strolling down the aisle of our local supermarkets. We no longer have to exert energy or "labor" to acquire our "fruits" or food.

Today we have a wide selection of food to tempt us. We are so wealthy compared to our ancestors! We not only have seemingly endless choices, we also have larger quantities of food available to us.

Worse yet, fast food provides affordable high calorie food choices that have become a staple of our diet, much to our detriment. Fast food is often the major source of nutrition in poor communities where supermarkets and healthier food choices are an expensive bus or cab ride away.

In rural areas, the labor involved in growing food has been greatly reduced by mechanization. Whereas farmers of 50 years ago were rarely overweight, it is now commonplace to see obesity reaching out to rural communities. Mechanization has progressed, but in many ways eating habits have not changed to adjust to a lower output of personal energy needed to acquire the food from the farm.

You can see where all of this is leading; we work less to obtain more food. What does that mean? It means we have become an obese society.

Our culture promotes overeating. With many families relying on two incomes, the trend is to "dine out" due to time constraints. Children raised 30 years ago were fortunate to receive a weekly allowance that permitted a rare trip to the local store for a small amount of candy. Children today often have access to disposable incomes that allow them daily access to fast food, candy and soft drinks outside of the family home and school. Prepared foods like fried chicken or pizza were once a major treat for a family, but have now become a regular part of our eating habit and sadly, they are often a part of the daily school lunch menu.

We have also become habitual consumers of junk food . I hesitate to call it "food," since these highly processed concoctions no longer resemble food that was harvested and eaten fresh just a century ago. We eat these products because we like them. Actually, we love them. We are addicted to them and we eat them not for survival, but for pleasure.

FOOD AS COMFORT

Eating satisfies our instinctive association between eating and survival. When you are genuinely hungry, eating makes you feel content and satisfied. That makes it easy to see why eating during times of emotional stress also relieves some of the emotional discomfort—or so we think. Stress makes us eat, binge eat and gorge even when we aren't hungry.

Addictive overeating happens to some people even when they aren't stressed. Food is a link in the positive feedback loop, where a behavior (eating) is rewarded by a positive emotion (comfort). Like Pavlov's dogs, we want to eat repetitively and excessively.

The recipe for an obese society is the lethal combination of sedentary jobs and couch potato time with the avalanche of junk food.

Again, like Pavlov's dogs, humans repeat certain behaviors over and over. Since we must eat to survive, it's not at all surprising that we have become food addicts: Food tastes good and so we eat it – and overdo it – over and over again. Overeating as an addiction is hard to kick, since we cannot give up on eating altogether.

RESETTING THE SOCIAL DEFINITION OF OBESITY

Our society has also developed a skewed view of what it means to be overweight. In the past, someone carrying an excess 20-30 pounds was generally seen as being overweight. Today people are more likely to think of a morbidly obese person—one who is 100 pounds overweight or more – as being overweight. If you fall into the "overweight" category, changes are that many people will perceive you as having a normal healthy weight.

Overweight individuals frequently have the same impression of their own weight - they falsely see themselves as having a normal weight.

How do you think of yourself? Find your place on the Body Mass Index (BMI) scale and get a reality check. One is available at: www.nhlbisupport. com/bmi

Another disturbing fact of modern life is that it has become common for children and teenagers to become obese. Young people rarely feel the physical effects of their excess weight. Although the current epidemic of Type 2 diabetes (once called adult onset diabetes) among children and teens shows the heavy toll being extracted by this terrible disease that may lead to heart disease by the time they're 40, kidney failure at 50, and death by 60.

As a teenager the excess weight has not had time to ravage their joints and cause arthritic pain. The youthful heart and lungs allow them to work and play without great limitation. They feel fine, so they don't believe their weight is an issue.

Celebrities are frequently overweight. Clothing styles often permit overweight people to dress fashionably and to disguise their weight.

The increasing prevalence of obesity has created a "new normal" of being overweight. When the majority of people are overweight or obese, it then becomes the "new normal." Lean, slender people become the exception and may even appear as "unhealthy" or "unattractive."

MEDICINE AND OBESITY

Modern medicine now has tools, mostly prescription drugs, which allow obese people to control the side effects of their excess weight without having to address their weight problems. If you are overweight, you can now take medication to control blood pressure, blood sugars and cholesterol. Although this is clearly an advance for science, it indirectly permits an obese person to stay overweight, as long as the diseases caused by excess weight are managed with medications.

When I was a full-time primary care doctor, I found it was easier to prescribe a medication than to counsel a patient on the need for weight loss. Prescription drug use also fosters a co-dependency between the patient and the doctor, as many drugs require regular monitoring for toxicity and this drives the need for further doctor visits.

As doctors, we have enabled patients to stay overweight, reassure them that their medical problem is controlled and indirectly give them permission to remain overweight. The resulting health care costs of obesity are enormous, not to mention the personal suffering that comes with a weight problem.

At the same time, until now, we have had little to offer an overweight person other than the expression, "eat less and exercise more." Now we can offer the OWL Diet that utilizes a LCD with appetite suppressants.

Morbid obesity may be managed by bariatric surgical procedures such as lap banding and gastric bypass to make the stomach smaller. Combined with a very low calorie intake of very selected foods, these surgeries have success stories of their own, but with the risks and costs associated with surgeries and hospital care.

It is somewhat ironic that as a medical profession we approve of low calorie intake for these surgical patients, yet if an obese person asks a primary care doctor about the safety of a low calorie diet like the OWL Diet, the response has typically been one of disapproval.

In my opinion, the world of science and medicine has failed to offer a viable weight loss plan to patients who are overweight to moderately obese. As a result, patients have sought out programs on their own and often undertake weight loss without medical supervision. The inability of the medical profession to service this need is perhaps compounded by the lack of insurance reimbursement for medical counseling, advice and supervision of weight loss programs.

As we move forward as a community, there is increasing awareness of the need for preventive medical services to be covered by health plans (private and government sponsored).

It only makes sense for overweight people to have access to programs that will help them lose weight, regain their health and prevent the serious (and expensive) health problems that are linked to obesity.

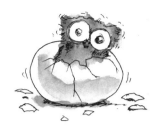

Chapter 4
THE BEGINNINGS OF
THE OWL DIET

Dr. A.T.W. Simeons is recognized as the physician who first combined a Very Low Calorie Diet (VLCD) of 500 calories per day with injections of the prescription hormone known as HCG. In the 1940s and 1950s, he ran a very successful weight loss facility in Rome, Italy.

His program was then, and is still today, an anecdotal program, meaning his HCG Diet has never undergone scientific scrutiny by large clinical trials. By clinical observation of his weight loss patients, he developed theories as to the mechanism of action of HCG when used in low doses for weight loss. His theories about HCG and how it works are just theories, unproven by science, but validated by the experiences of tens of thousands of patients.

It's ironic that Dr. Simeons and the popularity of his HCG diet faded from memory and the program that attracted attention decades ago seemed destined for the dustbin of weight loss schemes that have been forgotten.

Today's obesity pandemic has led many of us to look for a safe and effective way to lose pounds quickly. That desire, combined with the wealth of information available on the Internet, has led to a resurgence of interest in using HCG and low calorie dieting.

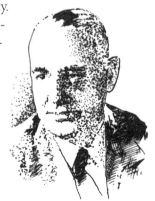

My years in medicine have taught me one truth: "The more you know, the less you know." After treating thousands of patients, an open-minded physician, as I believe myself to be, realizes how little we really understand about the workings of the human body. As we learn more about the complexities of bodily functions, the more we realize how much there is still to be learned.

I tell my patients that I do not know how HCG, when combined with my Low Calorie Diet (LCD), the OWL Diet, helps people to lose weight so quickly and easily. I do tell them that my experience has been that it is safe, and it does appear to be very effective. Any perceived risks of a calorie restricted diet have to be balanced against the enormous health risks of untreated obesity.

Do not undertake the use of HCG and the Low Calorie Diet (LCD) on your own. You need supervision by a licensed medical doctor with regular visits to his or her office. HCG is a prescription medication in the United States and is only legally available with a prescription.

THE OWL DIET TODAY

I have made many enhancements and changes to the original Simeons HCG Diet. Many of the beliefs that Dr. Simeons propagated more than six decades ago can be discredited, or at least challenged. My modern day program is simpler to understand and follow. As you will see, there are fewer "rules." I also have the safety of the public in mind, and I endorse a higher intake of calories per day to achieve that goal.

As a way of offering a clear message about these changes, I felt it was right to create a name for the new diet. I have chosen to name my program the Omaha Weight Loss Diet or OWL Diet for short.

The following paragraphs detail my differences from the Simeons Protocol, with my reasons for making these enhancements.

Food Choices and Frozen Foods

The original Simeons Protocol was based on a very limited selection of food items that were commonly available in Italy in the 1950s, when Dr. Simeons was in practice. I have added additional food selections in all four categories of meats, vegetables, fruits and beverages. We have also seen tremendous advancements in frozen foods, which can be safely incorporated into a modern protocol.

Sugar Substitutes

I permit the use of all sugar substitutes that are calorie free. Some critics point to studies that show that consumption of sugar substitutes has been associated with increased hunger, desire for sugar enhanced foods and increased risk for obesity. I agree that this may occur in some, but not all individuals.

Sugar substitutes are commonly used in diet soft drinks, iced teas and chewing gum. Use of these sugar free products represents food behaviors that are often well established by participants before they ever start the OWL Diet. For the purposes of compliance with the OWL Diet, the use of sugar substitutes is permitted. I do point out that, in the long run, I feel we should all limit our use of these products.

Some participants in my program report that they feel sugar substitutes are slowing their weight loss and that their progress is accelerated by stopping them. Once again, the variation between individuals and their response to sugar substitutes is by observation quite diverse. Each participant needs to tailor the use of these products based upon personal preference and the rate of weight loss.

Caffeine

Caffeine is permitted on the OWL Diet and is often consumed in tea, coffee or soft drinks. Once again, critics may challenge this notion. My observation is that caffeine can increase, decrease or have no effect on appetite. It varies by the individual. Many participants on the OWL Diet were using caffeine beverages before I see them and do not want to give them up. As a means of helping them succeed on the OWL Diet, I permit the use of caffeine. Stopping caffeine and starting a LCD can trigger problems with headaches in the first week of the program.

Low Calorie Diet (LCD)

I have adopted the term Low Calorie Diet (LCD) to describe the calorie intake permitted with the OWL Diet. The calorie intake will vary between participants based on their food selections for the day and whether or not they opt to have the one serving of an allowed alcoholic beverage in a given day. A variation in calories is most noticeable by the choice of lean beef over white chicken meat or white fish. The total calories permitted per day will range from 600 to 700.

As part of the LCD allowance, I permit up to 120 calories per day in the grain carbohydrates (a sizeable increase from the Simeons Protocol). Safety was my motivation for making this change. My observation of patients using the Simeons Very Low Calorie Diet (VLCD) of 500 calories per day was that they experienced excessive amounts of acidosis causing halitosis, headaches, muscle cramps and fatigue. With the LCD modification, patients feel better and have fewer effects from the acidosis of dieting and are therefore more likely to continue on the diet.

HCG Immunity

Simeons believed that patients would develop immunity to HCG. He advised the use of HCG for only six days per week and required intervals of time to be off HCG before restarting additional cycles.

I do not believe that immunity exists for the vast majority of participants. With the OWL Diet, I advise participants to use HCG daily for steady benefit and consistent results.

Continuous Monthly Cycles

Since we are not concerned about immunity and we now permit a higher intake of calories, I am able to offer monthly cycles of continuous HCG use. We see an average monthly weight loss of 15 pounds for women and 20 pounds for men.

Patients are safely permitted to continue monthly cycles "back to back" until they reach their weight loss goal. The momentum of successful weight loss is continued and patients learn to maintain lifelong behavioral changes towards healthier eating.

Vitamins and Supplements

This is a very important issue that will be addressed in Chapter 11. The OWL Diet is, by its very nature, low in food sources of calcium and supplementation with calcium is needed for most participants

You will also learn about the use of vitamin B-complex, B-12 injections, potassium, fiber and melatonin. The appropriate use of these supplements needs to be tailored to each participant based on their medical history and use of medications.

Creams, Oils and Cosmetics

The use of body creams, oils, lotions and cosmetics do not, in my experience, interfere with weight loss on the OWL Diet. They are permitted and this change from the Simeons Protocol is greatly appreciated by our patients! In the era of increasing risk of skin cancer from sun exposure, year round use of sun blocks is essential and highly recommended.

Menses

When women are menstruating, their hunger is frequently increased. I can find no logical explanation to withhold HCG based on the menstrual cycle in women. Daily use of HCG is encouraged, including during the menstrual period.

Fat is Fat

Dr. Simeons talked about "three kinds of fat," and theorized that during dieting, the body chooses certain fats to burn first. I do not follow that logic and my observation is that all fat stores are used as people are on the OWL program.

No Speculation About How HCG Works

Dr. Simeons had theories about how low dose HCG works. Since they remain unproven theories, I do not speculate on the mode of action of HCG. We simply do not know. What is more important to me is our observation that HCG does appear to help people lose weight on the OWL Diet.

No More Apple Days or Steak Days

Plateaus (no weight loss for a full two weeks despite complete adherence to the program) occur in any weight loss program.

Dr. Simeons attempted to break plateaus with either an "apple day" (eat nothing but five apples for a full day) or a "steak day" (do not eat all day, and then eat a large greasy steak in the evening).

I have attempted to use "apple days" and "steak days" with patients, and found them to be ineffective, misleading and counterintuitive. The best advice that I can offer is to stay committed and to look at the total accumulated weight loss. Plateaus cannot continue, due to the sheer arithmetic of following a LCD. Plateaus may be a sign that a weight loss participant needs to take a break from the LCD for at least one week and no more than four weeks, or the sign of an undiagnosed thyroid condition.

Salt Restriction

Dr. Simeons placed no restriction on salt, but today we know that excessive use of salt carries certain health risks. In a healthy individual, I permit the use of salt. If you have hypertension, coronary artery disease or heart failure, salt use should be limited.

Constipation

Constipation is a common challenge that we face with a LCD despite the high fiber content of the vegetables and fruits that you will be consuming.

Dr. Simeons did not intervene if patients only had a bowel movement every three to four days. My experience has been that constipation of three to four days' duration leads to retained weight, bloating, fatigue and risk of hemorrhoids. I prefer to advise the use of fiber to ensure a bowel pattern of once daily to every other day.

Massage

Massage is permitted, as there is no logical reason to withhold use of this very helpful service.

No More Phases

Dr. Simeons referred to "phases" during the HCG diet. I have found the use of this terminology to be confusing. The OWL Diet has three parts: fat loading, low calorie diet and maintenance.

PART II:

THE SPECIFICS OF THE OWL DIET

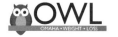

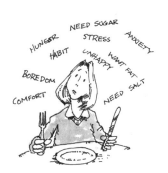

Chapter 5
CONTROLLING YOUR APPETITE

Hunger is a very complex mechanism of the human body. It is far more than simply not having eaten for several hours. Most of us eat for reasons well beyond survival. Hunger starts in your brain as positive memories of food triggers the desire to repeat the experience and satisfaction that comes from eating. Emotions surrounding the appearance, smell, taste and texture of food lead to physical cravings, that we call hunger.

Hunger may lead to eating because you are tired, stressed or feel like you deserve a reward - reasons that have little to do with your body's actual need for food.

Success with the OWL Diet requires strong commitment, focus and the willingness to sacrifice, even with the aid of HCG and other appetite suppressants.

Successful control of hunger and eating requires behavior changes in the following areas:

- Food available at home
- Food available at work
- Dining out
- Travel
- Social eating with friends and family
- Eating for comfort

But what makes the OWL Diet work is the use of prescription medicines that help control your hunger, making it possible for you to stay on the low calorie diet.

Without them, very few people would be able to stick with the rigors of the Low Calorie Diet (LCD). Medical science is working hard to address the dilemma of obesity and some advances are being made, particularly in the understanding of weight loss, long-term weight control, metabolism and the effects of exercise. I know we still have a lot to learn.

HCG

Human Chorionic Gonadotropin (HCG) is a hormone produced by pregnant women. HCG levels rise very quickly with pregnancy and the hormone is readily present in the urine of pregnant women. If you have ever used a home pregnancy test, then you have checked for the presence of HCG in your body.

Even though the combination of HCG with calorie restricted diets has been used worldwide for decades, the weight loss benefits have never been proven in any large significant placebo-controlled clinical trial.

In the United States, studies of that nature are required to be submitted to the Food and Drug Administration (FDA), before the government will approve the use of a prescription drug or hormone (like HCG) for a medical condition. HCG is produced by regulated pharmaceutical manufacturers in many countries, including the United States.

In America, the FDA has approved the use of HCG by injection to assist in stimulating ovulation. A pregnant woman may easily produce a million units of HCG per day. The FDA approved HCG dosage is often measured in thousands of units. When HCG is used at the low OWL Diet dose of 125-250 units daily, it will not interfere with birth control and will not raise a woman's fertility. Losing weight may increase fertility, but the small 125-250 IU daily injection of HCG will not on its own increase the risk of pregnancy. If pregnancy is not in your plans, you should continue to use a reliable form of birth control.

Since the FDA approved use of HCG has nothing to do with helping in weight loss, HCG for obesity is considered an "Off Label" use of the prescription hormone. Many drugs in America obtain FDA approval for one medical indication and then are found to be helpful for other conditions. The use of that drug or hormone is then considered "Off Label."

The OWL Diet currently uses a very low dose of 125-250 units of HCG administered by injection or transdermal cream every morning. At this low dose, I have not observed any adverse effects of the hormone.

Specifically, very low dose HCG does not:

- Cause men to grow breast tissue
- Affect moods in either men or women
- Affect sex drive

- Alter a woman's periods
- Raise her fertility
- Interfere with use of any forms of birth control
- Affect a man's voice
- Result in a change in body hair (either more hair or less hair)

As I say this, I'll note that losing weight is a stress on the body that can result in some temporary physical changes including causing irregular periods, loss of sleep or changes in hair growth.

The benefit of low dose HCG is observed to be:

- Appetite suppression
- The direction of fat burning when combined with a calorie restricted diet

The FDA says HCG should not be used in men with a history of prostate or testicular cancer.

The OWL Diet is not recommended for anyone under 21, women who are pregnant, breast-feeding or planning on becoming pregnant in the near future.

HOW HCG WORKS

The ways the hormone HCG may help in weight loss are not known. Any discussion to the contrary is speculation or theory. As a result, the FDA correctly states that "HCG has not been demonstrated to be effective adjunctive therapy in the treatment of obesity, there is no substantial evidence that it increases weight loss beyond that resulting from caloric restriction, that it causes a more attractive or normal distribution of fat, or that it decreases the hunger and discomfort associated with calorie-restricted diet."

I agree with the FDA statement, since there is no scientific proof regarding the use of HCG and dieting. The use of HCG for weight loss is anecdotal, meaning it is based on case histories and personal experience rather than scientific research.

My statements about the use of HCG and weight loss are based on my personal observations and are echoed by hundreds of my patients who have followed the OWL Diet, lost weight and have improved their overall health and well being.

I also agree with the medical and scientific community that obesity is a huge medical problem in our society and that the personal and financial costs of obesity are monumental. The government also recognizes the impact that obesity is having upon our nation.

HCG INJECTIONS

First of all, it is important to understand that the absorption of orally swallowed HCG is so low that it should be considered as completely ineffective. Taking HCG in a liquid or solid form that is swallowed is not a viable option.

Second, "homeopathic HCG" as now available for sale on the Internet is not therapeutic. The dose is too small and it is therefore a placebo.

The "gold standard" for administering HCG is to do so by injection. Injection is the route that I personally used to lose my weight.

HCG for injection is sold as a sterile powder in glass vials. The powder is reconstituted with bacteriostatic water, and the solution is then stable for 60 days when refrigerated.

The standard dose of HCG by injection is 125 IU (international units) administered IM (intramuscular), once every morning, seven days per week for four continuous weeks (one cycle).

At my med spa, I reconstitute the HCG and perform a dilution with the result that 0.5cc equals a dose of 125 IU. I prefer to pre-fill the syringes for our patients. Every week when they see us, patients receive a bag of seven pre-filled syringes. We use the 3cc syringe and 25G needle that is 5/8" long. The injection is nearly painless and my patients learn to administer it to themselves very easily. I've found the easiest technique for HCG shots is as follows:

1. Your skin at the injection site should be clean and free of lotion or cream.
2. Wash your hands thoroughly with soap and warm water.
3. Sit on a chair or on the side of the bed with your feet flat on the floor.
4. Use a single alcohol prep pad to clean your skin on the front (top) of your thigh or on the outer side of your thigh, over the large muscle, the quadriceps.
5. Use a cotton ball to dry the alcohol. (This reduces the discomfort).
6. Hold the needle in your hand like a pen or dart.
7. Carefully remove the cap covering the needle, taking care not to touch the needle.
8. With your hand six inches from the thigh, point the needle at a 90 degree angle (perpendicular) to the skin. Use a wrist action, and

with one smooth motion confidently place the needle into the muscle. The discomfort should be minimal. If there is pain on insertion, the needle may be withdrawn and placed into another location.

9. Holding the syringe with both hands, carefully pull back slightly on the plunger. If blood appears in the clear HCG fluid, you're in a vein, and the needle should be removed without injection and placed into an alternate location.

10. Once you are satisfied you're not in a vein, inject the HCG slowly, taking about 5 seconds to empty the syringe.

11. Leave the needle in the thigh for another 5 to 10 seconds to allow the fluid to absorb.

12. Remove the needle from your thigh. Do not recap the needle onto the syringe. Discard the needle and syringe, attached to each other, into a suitable biohazard sharps container. Sharps containers are available from your physician or pharmacist.

13. Apply light pressure with the cotton ball and use a plastic bandage if needed.

The risks of injection include discomfort, bruising or development of skin infection at the injection site. Although self-injection may initially seem complicated to the uninitiated, the technique is simple and quickly learned.

I always have each patient receive training in self-injection as part of the initial consultation before beginning the OWL Diet. My rule is that you have to show me that you can safely administer a practice dose before leaving the med spa with your supply of HCG.

HCG CREAM

I've used HCG cream with very good results in my OWL Diet patients.

The notion of applying cream to the skin as an acceptable means of delivering hormones to the body is certainly not a new one. In modern medicine, there are numerous examples of FDA approved transdermal products that deliver hormones for contraception, postmenopausal hormone replacement therapy and testosterone deficiency. Transdermal absorption of hormones is clearly well documented and efficient.

That fact made it easy for me to embrace the notion that application of cream containing HCG would be effective and safe. The technique is simple.

Cream is applied in a dose of 125 IU once per day (same dose as with injection) as follows:

1. Wash and dry your skin.
2. The simplest choice for men and women alike is to apply a measured dose of the cream to the inner forearm.
3. Remove watches and bracelets.
4. Apply the measured dose of HCG cream to one inner forearm. Then rub both forearms together until the cream is absorbed (about one minute). Avoid putting other cream, lotion or sunscreen on this area for one hour.
5. Other skin locations that are acceptable to use are the female breast and inner thighs.
6. Men should avoid hairy areas, and as a result the inner forearm is often the best choice.

SUBLINGUAL HCG

HCG has also been administered by the sublingual (under the tongue) method. In modern medicine, we often use the sublingual method of drug delivery for select medications (nitroglycerin heart medication, for example).

The technique for using the sublingual method is to place a small tablet under the tongue. The tablet needs to dissolve quickly, and is then absorbed by the blood vessels under the tongue. Once absorbed, the medication is rapidly spread throughout the body.

To use the sublingual method with HCG, a pharmacist takes a measured amount of HCG powder and dissolves it in sterile water (use of an artificial sweetener is optional). The solution is placed in a glass bottle with a calibrated dropper, and is stored in the refrigerator. There is no powder or tablet form of HCG that exists today that is effective when placed under the tongue, or swallowed.

When sublingual HCG solution is placed under the tongue, it must be held there for at least three minutes. The hope is that the HCG will diffuse out of the solution and be absorbed by the veins under the tongue. Unfortunately, the liquid itself is not absorbed. I found that over the course of waiting three minutes, saliva combines with the HCG solution, and increases the overall volume of fluid held under the tongue.

After three minutes, the HCG solution is removed from the mouth by spitting it out. Swallowing would not offer any additional benefit. Sublingual HCG solution is often taken twice per day for a total daily dose of 250 IU per day. I suspect the practice of dosing the HCG solution twice a day has evolved due to the poor absorption of the sublingual method.

My opinion is that sublingual HCG is cumbersome and inconvenient. Furthermore, in my experience, approximately half of all sublingual HCG users reported poor control of hunger, suggesting that the absorption was either very poor or none at all. As a result, I no longer recommend the use of sublingual HCG drops or solution.

PHENTERMINE

Some OWL Diet participants combine HCG with another prescription medication, the appetite suppressant phentermine. In the US, phentermine is FDA approved and is available by prescription from a pharmacy.

Your doctor should be aware of the prescribing recommendations for phentermine and follow them. As of the writing of this book, insurance companies in the US do not generally reimburse patients for phentermine prescriptions. It is available in generic form, and is not considered to be expensive (generally less than a dollar a day).

Currently, the two most common dosage forms are 15 mg. and 37.5 mg. Both strengths are in tablet form and are easy to swallow.

Examples of dosing schedules that I have used are:

- 15 mg. - 1 taken first thing in the morning with an additional optional dose of one taken at noon
- 37.5 mg. - 1/2 to 1 tablet taken every morning

The most common side effect of phentermine is dry mouth, but it may also cause insomnia, anxiety, palpitations or raise blood pressure. Because of the potential side effects, it is not recommended for everyone and phentermine use requires medical supervision. Unlike HCG, the appetite suppressing effect of phentermine often seems to decline after about two months; so breaks from taking the medication are often needed.

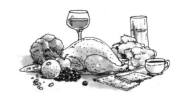

Chapter 6
THE OWL DIET

I suggest you read this entire book and do some careful planning before starting the OWL Diet.

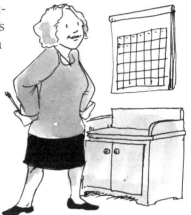

The food choices are very specific. Being organized will help to ensure success. It's probably not a good idea to start when you are also planning a vacation or travel associated with business.

Here is the OWL Diet Plan. For the first month you'll need to adhere to it without exceptions. Later in the process, you will have the option of some "tweaks," or modifications that usually work (see Chapter 8) and give you a little more food variety.

FAT LOADING

The first day that you start taking HCG is Day One of the OWL Diet. On Day One and Day Two, you will "fat load." During these two days, you will eat foods that are high in fat content. Consider these your last two days of eating food that will from this point forward be categorized as unhealthy and undesirable.

Why do we recommend that people fat load? The original Simeons Protocol provided for fat loading. I don't really know why this technique helps people to lose more weight the first week, but based on my own experience and the experience of my patients, it does work to jump start weight loss.

Dr. Simeons speculated on the mechanism, but it is an opinion that has not been validated. Fat loading is unscientific and anecdotal. It is however great fun for some individuals!

What I can tell you is this: I have observed that the people who "fat load" do in fact lose more weight in the first week. As you consume these fatty foods, please keep in mind that if you overindulge in fat rich foods and gain weight during fat loading, I do not give you credit for that additional weight. Your starting weight is taken from your initial consultation or visit. You will need to lose any weight gained from fat loading to get back to your starting weight, and then lose additional pounds for the remainder of the week, leading up to your Week One follow-up visit.

As a physician, I certainly struggled at first with the notion of fat loading. The advice seemed to appear counterintuitive to a weight loss program. However, having seen it in action, I can attest to its apparent effectiveness.

What if you refuse to fat load or simply choose not to? Will this sabotage the program? The answer is "no," but your weight loss the first week may be less than others who fat load.

What if you have a medical condition that might be compromised by two days of eating fat-rich foods?

OWL Diet Foods to be Consumed Daily:

- *Water: 2 quarts, at least*
- *Meat: 7 ounces*
- *Vegetables: 4 cups*
- *Fruit: 2 servings*
- *Fresh Salad Greens, Spinach, Celery: unlimited*
- *Grain Carbohydrates: 100 calories*

Optional:

- *Coffee, tea, diet sodas or other calorie-free drinks*
- *Alcoholic beverages – 1 drink per day, maximum (100 calories per day)*

One example would be diabetes mellitus, which could cause an unsafe rise in blood sugar from the increased fat caloric intake. In this case, fat loading should be moderated, with attention made to careful monitoring of your blood sugar at home. A mild increase in blood sugar for two days should not cause adverse effects. If concern persists, then skip fat loading altogether.

If you have heart disease, it would probably be best to skip the fat loading days since studies have shown that even one large fatty meal can put the heart at risk for strain and could potentially trigger chest pain (angina), or a heart attack (acute coronary syndrome).

If you take a break from the HCG program, and then restart less than one month later, do not repeat fat loading. If however, more than a month has passed, then a repeat of fat loading does seem to be reasonable, but is by no means mandatory.

What food selection meets the criteria for fat loading? I almost hate to mention these foods, but they would include fast food such as hamburger and fries, potato chips, deep fried foods (battered fish), ice cream, pizza, pastries and donuts. The list is in fact endless, as there is no shortage of unhealthy fat rich foods in our culture from which to choose. Other healthier options would include pasta with extra olive oil, cheese, salmon and cream with coffee.

BEVERAGES

The most important message here is to drink lots of water. A half a gallon - 68 oz. (2 liters) is the minimum and more is better. Water is consumed by the body during the course of burning fat calories. In addition, water intake is vital to the ability of the kidneys and to produce an adequate output of urine. Water also helps curb your appetite and maintain your energy. Drink water to help lose weight, and drink plenty of water for a healthy life.

On the OWL Diet, your pattern of bowel movements may change. It is not unusual for a person who normally reports one or two stools per day to notice a change to less than one stool per day. Maintaining an adequate intake of fluid will reduce the risk of constipation.

Milk and cream are **not** permitted. In fact, you will not be permitted to use any dairy products while on the OWL Diet. That includes all cheeses and yogurts. It is not that dairy products are unhealthy or bad for you. I feel that the caloric allowance of the LCD is best spent on consuming fresh fruits, meats, vegetables and grain carbohydrates.

You can drink coffee and tea during the OWL Diet in both hot and cold forms. I do permit the use of caffeine. Some people find that caffeine stimulates appetite. If this is the case for you, try to go caffeine-free or taper down your use of caffeine. Going from several caffeine containing beverages per day to none can trigger headaches and anxiety, so use your best judgment.

Any beverage that contains caffeine will have a diuretic effect on the kidney, meaning that it will trigger the production of urine. As a result, you may lose as much water through the urine as you take in with the caffeinated beverage. Caffeinated beverages therefore do not count towards the minimum 2 liters of water intake.

I do permit the use of all artificial sweeteners, including the brand names Sweet-N-Low, Equal, Splenda, Truvia and Stevia. Non-dairy creamers are not calorie free, and are not allowed.

Soft drinks (sodas and pops) are not a healthy beverage selection in general, due to their lack of nutritional value and high phosphate content. Soft drink consumption, however, can be habit forming, so I don't advise you to change your consumption of soft drinks while you are on the HCG diet. Of course, you must choose diet or zero-calorie soft drinks. Once you have achieved your weight loss goal, I strongly urge you to reassess your soft drink consumption and wean yourself away from them.

There are now many flavored beverages that are also calorie free. I permit the use of any of these products. Be sure to carefully read the product label to confirm the absence of calories.

Alcohol use will be dealt with separately at the end of this chapter.

OWL MEATS

Your meat is weighed before it is cooked. You are permitted 7 oz. (200 grams) of meat per day. After you cook the meat, divide it into two meals, so that you are having 3.5 oz. at lunch and 3.5 oz. at supper. By dividing your meat into two meals, you will have better hunger control, better energy and a better fat burn.

Alternatively, you may have your entire daily meat allowance of 7 oz. (200 grams) at one meal. If you follow a once daily format, and are not losing weight at a rate of three to four pounds per week, then you will need to change to 3.5 oz. twice a day. Some people prefer to graze on their 7 oz. meat allowance over the course of the day, and this seems to work out just fine.

You will need a basic food scale to weigh your meat portions. A simple spring scale with a basket on top will suffice and can be purchased at many larger department stores or online. As of the writing of this book, the scale should not cost more than $10.

Your meat is prepared without cooking oil. This means that using nonstick pans, grilling, broiling and baking in the oven are good choices for meat preparation. Poaching and boiling are also acceptable. There are non-stick cooking sprays that are rated as zero calories that may be used. Always check the labels before using a product to ensure zero-calorie content.

Meats may be purchased fresh or frozen. Frozen foods may not have any additional oil, breading, sauce or other additives with calories. You will have to cook your meat. One exception to the "cook your own meat" rule is shrimp, which is often sold pink in color and ready to eat. That type of shrimp is fine, as it has only been steamed, or you may buy your shrimp raw and cook it yourself. Avoid precooked meats (such as chicken), canned meats, cold cuts or preserved meats.

You must consume your 7 oz. allowance of meat every day – no more and no less. Meat protein is an important part of the fat burning process with the OWL Diet. You may mix your variety of meats eaten in a given day, for example by having 3.5 oz. of chicken at lunch, and 3.5 oz. of white fish for supper.

Choose from this list of meats every day:

- **Chicken:** You must buy uncooked chicken meat that is fresh or frozen from fresh. Pre-cooked is not permitted, nor are chicken cold cuts or other processed forms.

  Choose white chicken breasts or chicken tenders (tenderloins). Thighs, wings or other brown meat are *not* permitted. The white chicken meat must be free of fat and skin before cooking.

  You may pre-cook chicken at home, place it in 3.5 oz. portions and store it in the refrigerator in plastic bags. Chicken may then be re-warmed or eaten cold. Dicing chicken will make it appear to go further and is a great addition to salads, vegetables and homemade soup.

- **Beef:** For steaks, you may choose from sirloin steak or filet mignon, as long as all visible fat is removed. Bacon wrapping of the steak is *not* permitted.

  For ground beef, ask the butcher to grind sirloin steak, or choose the leanest form of ground beef that is available. Small 3.5 oz. patties may be grilled and also bake well in the oven.

  Beef tenderloin is also acceptable, but typically is much more expensive. Kobe beef is *not* permitted.

Limit your consumption of beef to twice per week since 7 oz. of lean steak is approximately twice the calories of white chicken or white fish.

- **Bison and Venison:** Bison and venison are considered lean, but you must still be very careful. If you choose to use a ground game meat, it must not have any visible particles of fat. Steak must not have any visible marbling.
- **Shrimp and Scallops:** You may use shrimp that is fresh or frozen. Shrimp is the one exception to the statement that you must cook all of your own meat. It is often sold precooked by steaming, is pink in color and is acceptable. Scallops are an alternative.

  You may *not* use any other shellfish (such as lobster or crab).
- **White Fish:** White fish may be purchased fresh or fresh frozen, but once again you must cook the fish yourself. Choose from: Tilapia, Sole, Orange roughy, Halibut, Perch, or Cod.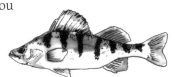

  You may *not* have tuna, ahi or salmon.

OWL VEGETABLES

If you like vegetables, you will like the OWL Diet. I allow a large variety of vegetables and encourage you to mix and match with them during a meal and over the course of a day.

Salads are a great way to stay full with my diet. *I permit unlimited amounts of fresh salad greens, spinach and celery.* The calorie count is so small, that I consider this "free food"! Most OWL Dieters make a large salad for lunch and supper to combine with their meat allowance, and a variety of cooked vegetables. That way, you have two very significant meals per day, at lunch and supper, to enjoy.

You may use fresh lemon or lime juice as well as a variety of vinegars on your salads. Walden Farms is a brand of flavored salad dressings that are calorie free, but do use additives and sucralose (Learn more about the entire line of Walden Farms products at: www.waldenfarms.com).

All other vegetables are limited to 4 cups of uncooked diced or cut vegetables per day. Vegetables must be fresh or fresh frozen. They may be cooked or eaten raw.

Choose 4 cups daily from this list of approved vegetables:

- Onions, all varieties
- Peppers, all varieties and colors, sweet or hot
- Mushrooms
- Radishes
- Tomatoes (counted as a vegetable, not a fruit)
- Green beans
- Cucumbers
- Dill pickles
- Summer squash
- Zucchini
- Winter squash (acorn, ace, spaghetti, to name a few)
- Broccoli
- Cauliflower
- Asparagus (great added cold to salads)
- Cabbage
- Brussel Sprouts
- Sprouts
- Snow Peas (limit of 1/2 cup per day)

You may **not** have:

- Canned vegetables
- Corn
- Carrots
- Shelled peas
- Potatoes
- Sweet potatoes

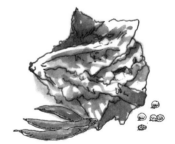

OWL FRUITS

You are permitted 2 servings of fresh or frozen fruit per day. Eat fruit to start the day, as a snack between meals or in the evening.

Choose from the following fruits, listed as a single serving size:

- 1 apple (any color)
- 1 orange

- 1/3 cup blueberries
- 6 medium-sized strawberries
- 2 cups of any melon, such as cantaloupe or watermelon (limit of 1 serving per day from melons)
- 1/2 grapefruit (Grapefruit may interfere with the metabolism of many medications, so check with your doctor.)

You may **not** have:

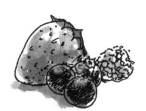

- Canned or dried fruits
- Bananas
- Pineapple
- Mango
- Grapes

OWL GRAIN CARBOHYDRATES

One of the following is permitted per day. I have mentioned actual brand names available in the United States, but other brands may be considered. The total calorie content permitted per day with these grain source carbohydrates is in the range of 80-120 calories, with no more than 15 calories from fat.

Although it is tempting to use these with lunch and supper, they are best divided into 2-4 servings, and used in the same way as they fruit – at the start of the day, as a snack and in the evenings.

Choose from the following list:

- Italian breadsticks made by the "Grissini method" - 4 pieces per day (Alessi brand sesame or garlic breadsticks)
- Melba toast - 5 pieces per day (Traditional rectangular - London brand of classic, wheat, rye and sesame)
- Crisp Breads – 2 pieces per day (Swedish or German - Wasa brand)
- Sesame cracker - 4 individual crackers per day (Ak-Mak brand)
- Mini Bag of Microwaveable Popcorn 94% fat-free - 1 bag per day (Orville Redenbacker's Smart Pop)
- Thin Sandwich Rolls (various brands) - 1 roll per day
- Some versions of pita pockets (as low as 80 calories per pocket) - 1 per day (Kangaroo Brand Sandwich Multi-Grain Pocket)
- Bagel Thins – 1 per day (Thomas' brand)

The grain carbohydrates are best used between meals when a snack is desired, since the crunchiness will give you satisfaction. Another option is to crumble them and make a topping for chicken or fish, or simply add to a salad.

The following are *not* permitted:

- Pasta
- Rice
- Regular bread
- Beans (baked, black, kidney or other)

OWL FATS AND OILS

This is the easiest area to cover since none are allowed. *You may not use oils of any kind.*

In the United States, all forms of PAM brand non-stick cooking sprays are rated as zero calorie and may be used. Note that most of these products will say a 1/3-second spray is zero calories.

There are products that offer a buttery flavor, but they are not dairy sourced and are also zero calorie. An example is the soy-derived sprays under the brand names "Smart Balance" or "I Can't Believe It's Not Butter." Only the spray forms of these brands are permitted. The product sold in tubs is different, is not calorie, and is not approved with the OWL Diet. Be careful to read product labels to make sure that it is in fact rated as calorie-free and only then may it be used on food.

OWL SEASONINGS

You are allowed the fresh or bottled juice of lemons and limes. If you're using bottled juices, be sure the product is rated zero calorie. The juice of each fresh lime or lemon is approximately 10 calories, so limit yourself to two per day.

Lemon and lime juice can be used to add flavor to chicken, fish and salads. You may also use lemon juice with water and artificial sweetener for a refreshing lemonade, or added to teas.

The following are allowed:

- Salt (limit your use if you have high blood pressure, ankle swelling or heart disease).
- Pepper
- Salt substitutes (Mrs. Dash's brand is one example)

- Fresh or dried herbs
- Garlic
- Ginger
- Cinnamon
- Curry
- Virtually any other dried spice
- Hot sauce (Tabasco or Cholula brand names, for example)
- Traditional yellow mustard (French's brand)
- Worcestershire sauce
- Bragg's Liquid Aminos (calorie free soy sauce)

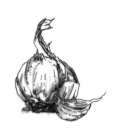

If you enjoy spices, then I encourage you to season and spice up your food.

The following are **not** permitted:

- Ketchup (You can make your own salsa by dicing up tomatoes, onion, fresh cilantro and adding lemon juice.)
- Barbeque sauce
- Mayonnaise
- Marinades or salad dressings that are not rated zero calorie

ALCOHOL

I have often been challenged, and even criticized, for allowing alcohol consumption during the OWL Diet.

My rationale is simple. If no alcohol is allowed on the diet and a person "cheats" and has a drink, feelings of shame, guilt and failure may develop. This may lead a person to quit the diet altogether, or cheat so much on alcohol that the weight loss program is truly sabotaged. By allowing alcohol use, I'm recognizing that the social use of alcohol in our society is common and readily accepted as a normal part of life.

When I allow one alcoholic beverage per day, I'm also able to set guidelines as to what choices are acceptable. My allowance is the equivalent of up to 100 calories per day, and the choices allowed are very specific.

If you choose not to have an alcoholic beverage on a given day, then the policy is "Have it or lose it." In other words, you cannot "bank it up" by not drinking for several days and then having several on a Saturday night, or use those 100 calories elsewhere in your food intake.

Choose from one of the following, per day:

- **Wine:** A 4 oz. pour of dry white or red wine. Grape varieties that are dry include: Sauvignon Blanc, Pinot Grigio, Pinot Noir, Chardonnay, Cabernet, Cabernet Sauvignon, Merlot, Red Zinfandel and Shiraz.
- **Beer:** light (up to 100 calories)
- **Liquor:** 1 1/2 oz. of liquor such as vodka, gin, whiskey, bourbon or scotch - may be mixed with water or a diet soft drink.

You may *not* have:

- Sweet wines - such as Port, Sherry, Pink Zinfandel, or dessert wines
- Any mixers that are not zero calories
- Brandy or cognac

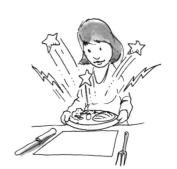

Chapter 7
OWL DIET
MEAL PLANS

Now you know what foods to choose from. With a little creativity, you can create flavorful meals that will keep you on track and keep your taste buds happy. That's good news considering that boredom with food choice is one of the top reasons for people to quit any diet.

Look at the following meal plans as a framework to help stimulate your own ideas on how to mix and match the allowed foods. Each of us has different food likes and dislikes. Customize the OWL Diet to meet your own personal preferences. I also want you to challenge yourself to try some new foods, or revisit foods that you may have categorized in the past as foods that you did not like. Our taste buds change with time and you may find some new positive food experiences!

Choose a variety of vegetables, fruits and meats to enjoy. This will satisfy your craving for food variety and provide a mix of higher and lower calorie foods.

Although I do not ask you to count calories per day, some OWL Diet participants find it helpful to obtain a calorie counting book or use a free on-line resource for calorie counting. On most days, you will average approximately 600-700 calories. On a day that you choose a lean beef steak, your daily calorie count may well reach 800 calories. Limit beef to once or twice per week and on days that you have steak, choose lower calorie fruit such as grapefruit and blueberries.

The following meal plans do not mention specifics of how you will cook your meats and vegetables. I leave that up to your own creativity based on individual cooking and seasoning preferences. The recipe section in Chapter 10 will surely tweak your creativity.

Remember that all forms of PAM brand sprays are zero calorie and that you will not use any other forms of cooking oils. Indoor grilling with non-stick pans and George Foreman grills are popular, as is outdoor grilling. Also try poaching your fish and chicken. The oven bake method works well for all forms of meat and many of the vegetables.

Some of the following meal plans include one drink of alcohol. You are allowed one drink per day from the approved list, but remember you can't "bank up" your drinks. In other words, have one drink per day, or lose it. By avoiding alcohol altogether, you will lose weight faster. With all of the plans, remember that you should drink a minimum of 68 oz. (2 liters) of water per day.

For each meal plan, the choices from each major food category are listed. This is followed by a suggested way of combining the food choices over the course of the day. Calories are estimated and placed in parentheses after each food or beverage listed. Celery and salad greens add small but nominal amounts of additional calories that I have not included in the overall calorie count. Remember you can eat these freely.

At the end of each day, you'll see an estimate of the total calories consumed.

Other low calorie snacks may be added such as:

- 3 pickled banana peppers (10 calories)
- Vlasic "No Sugar Added" pickles – 3 small gherkins (5 calories) or 1 bread & butter dill spear (7 calories)
- Celery

For condiments try:

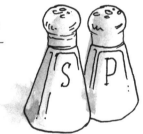

- Zero-calorie traditional yellow mustard like French's and hot spicy sauces such as Cholula or Tabasco
- Sugar-free jams or jellies like Smucker's or Polaner (10 calories per serving size of 1 Tbsp.) that combine well with Ak-Mak crackers or Melba Toast

Prepare your food in advance of most meals. By being organized, you are able to stay focused and on track with the OWL Diet.

If you have to "cheat" and eat extra calories, always choose from foods that are approved on the diet.

SAMPLE MEAL PLAN

Day One

    Vegetables: 6 Brussel sprouts (45), 1 cup of sliced green cabbage (18), 1 cup of asparagus (46), 1 cup of cauliflower (20)
    Meat: 3.5 oz. lean bison steak (142), 3.5 oz. cod (82)
    Fruit: 2 apples (72 ea.)
    Grain Carbs: 1 mini bagel (110)
    Total Calories for the Day = 607

    Breakfast: 1/2 toasted mini bagel with zero-calorie Smart Balance spray, water, black coffee
    Mid-morning snack: 1/2 apple, water
    Lunch: 3.5 oz. cod, 6 Brussel sprouts, 1 cup of asparagus, fresh spinach, rice vinegar, green tea, water
    Afternoon snack: celery, calorie-free dill pickle, water
    Dinner: 3.5 oz. lean bison steak, 1 cup cauliflower, 1 cup sliced green cabbage, leaf lettuce salad with Walden Farm dressing, green tea, water, 1/2 apple
    Evening snack: 1/2 toasted mini bagel, 1 apple, water

Day Two

    Vegetables: 2 cups green beans (68), 1/2 cup diced onion (47), 1 medium red tomato (48), 1 green pepper (20)
    Meat: 7 oz. white chicken (332)
    Fruit: 2 tangerines (45 ea.)
    Grain Carbs: 1 thin sandwich (100)
    Total Calories for the Day = 705

    Breakfast: 1 tangerine, coffee with Splenda, water
    Mid-morning snack: celery, water
    Lunch: 3.5 oz. white chicken on 1/2 thin sandwich with 1/2 diced tomato, lettuce, 1/2 green pepper, Walden Farm dressing, 1 cup green beans, Earl Grey tea with RealLemon, water
    Afternoon snack: celery, coffee with sugar free-Torani flavoring, water
    Dinner: 3.5 oz. white chicken on 1/2 thin sandwich with 1/2 diced tomato, spinach, 1/2 green pepper, 1 cup green beans, red wine vinegar, Mrs. Dash, pepper, herbal tea, water
    Evening snack: 1 tangerine, water

Day Three

Vegetables: 1 green pepper (20), 1 cup sliced cucumber (14), 2 cups tomato (96)

Meat: 7 oz. 95% lean ground beef (324)

Fruit: 1 cup strawberries (45), 1/3 cup blueberries (27)

Grain Carbs: 1 Kangaroo brand whole wheat pita pocket (80)

Alcohol: 1 Bud Select beer (55)

Total Calories for the Day = 661

Breakfast: 1/2 cup strawberries with Truvia, black coffee, water

Mid-morning snack: 1/2 cup sliced cucumber with Walden Farm dressing, celery, SoBe zero-calorie drink

Lunch: 3.5 oz. patty of lean ground beef, 1/2 green pepper, 1 cup diced tomato, Bragg's Liquid Aminos for seasoning, romaine lettuce, coffee, water

Afternoon snack: 1/2 cup of strawberries with Truvia, diet soda, water

Dinner: 3.5 oz. lean ground beef in whole wheat pita pocket, with 1/2 cup sliced cucumber, 1/2 green pepper, 1 cup diced tomato, romaine lettuce, Walden Farm's dressing, Bud Select beer, water

Evening snack: 1/3 cup blueberries, water

Day Four

Vegetables: 1 cup asparagus (46), 1 cup green beans (34), 1/2 cup mushrooms (19), 1/2 cup onions (47), 1 green pepper (20), 1/2 cup cabbage (9)

Meat: 3.5 oz. filet mignon beef steak trimmed fat-free (216), 3.5 oz. cod fish (82)

Fruit: 2 cups cantaloupe (114), 1/3 cup blueberries (27)

Grain Carbs: 1 Kangaroo brand whole wheat pita pocket (80)

Total Calories for the Day = 694

Breakfast: 1 cup cantaloupe, diet cola, water

Mid-morning snack: celery, 1/2 cup raw green peppers, water

Lunch: 3.5 oz. cod, 1 cup asparagus, 1/2 green pepper, endive, 1/2 cup onions, tea, water

Afternoon snack: 1/3 cup blueberries with Equal sweetener

Dinner: 3.5 oz. filet mignon beef steak, 1/2 cup mushrooms, Worcestershire sauce, whole wheat pita pocket, 1 cup green beans, 1/2 cup of cabbage, iceberg lettuce, water

Evening snack: 1 cup cantaloupe, water

Day Five

Vegetables: 1/2 cup mushrooms (19), 1/2 cup chopped onions (47), 1 cup green beans (34), 1/2 cup snap peas (30), 1 cup asparagus (46), 1/2 cup sliced cucumber (7)

Meat: 3.5 oz. white chicken meat (166), 3.5 oz. tilapia fish (99)

Fruit: 1 orange (65), 2 cups watermelon (100)

Grain Carbs: 5 Melba toast (95)

Total Calories for the Day = 708

Breakfast: 2 slices of Melba toast, black coffee, water

Mid-morning snack: 1 orange, 1 slice Melba toast, water

Lunch: 3.5 oz. chicken, lettuce, 1/2 cup sliced cucumber, 1/2 cup snap peas, 1 cup green beans, water

Afternoon snack: 1 cup watermelon, 1 slice Melba toast, diet soda, water

Dinner: 3.5 oz. tilapia, lettuce, 1/2 cup mushrooms, 1/2 cup chopped onions, 1 cup asparagus, water, sugar free iced tea.

Evening snack: 1 cup watermelon, 1 slice Melba toast, water

Day Six

Vegetables: 1 cup snap peas (60), 1 cup banana peppers (33), 1 green pepper (20), 1 cup cauliflower (20)

Meat: 7 oz. halibut fish (217)

Fruit: 1 full grapefruit (74)

Grain Carbs: 4 Alessi garlic Italian breadsticks (120)

Alcohol: 4 oz. dry wine (95)

Total Calories for the Day = 639

Breakfast: 1/2 grapefruit, water, black coffee

Mid-morning snack: 1 breadstick, water

Lunch: 3.5 oz. halibut, 1/2 cup snap peas, 1/2 cup banana peppers, 1/2 green pepper, 1/2 cup cauliflower, salad greens, water

Afternoon snack: 1 breadstick, diet soda, water

Dinner: 3.5 oz. halibut, 1/2 cup snap peas, 1/2 cup banana peppers, 1/2 green pepper, 1/2 cup cauliflower, salad greens, dry wine

Evening snack: 1/2 grapefruit, 2 breadsticks

Day Seven

Vegetables: 6 pieces Brussel sprouts (45), 1/2 cup shredded green cabbage(9), 1 cup sliced cucumber(14), 1 green pepper (20), 1 cup cauliflower(20)

Meat: 3.5 oz. shrimp (100), 3.5 oz. scallops (118)

Fruit: 2 medium apples (72 ea.)

Grain Carbs: "100 Calorie" mini-bag microwave popcorn (100)

Alcohol: 1.5 oz. vodka with diet tonic water (97)

Total Calories for the Day = 667

Breakfast: water, black coffee

Mid-morning snack: 1 apple with Walden Farms caramel dip, water, coffee

Lunch: 3.5 oz. shrimp on lettuce salad, 1/2 green pepper, RealLime, seasonings, 1 cup cauliflower, water

Afternoon snack: 1/2 bag of popcorn, water

Dinner: 3.5 oz. scallops, 1/2 green pepper, 1/2 cup cabbage, 6 Brussel sprouts, 1 cup sliced cucumber on lettuce, tea, water

Evening snack: vodka with diet tonic water, 1 apple, 1/2 bag of popcorn

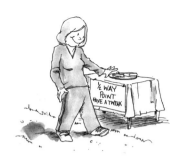

Chapter 8
TWEAKS

After you've been on the OWL Diet for a full month, or you have reached the halfway point toward your goal weight, you and your taste buds may need a boost. Good news! Now you are allowed a few "Tweaks" that will help keep you on track with losing more weight, and getting to your goal.

"Tweaks" are foods you can add to the OWL Diet, that based on their calorie and fat content should be acceptable alternatives. I don't allow Tweaks to be used at the start of the diet because: *Tweaks sometimes slow the rate of weight loss.*

In addition, I have found that if there are too many food choices at the outset, there can be confusion over what foods are allowed and how to combine them over the course of a given day.

It is great fun to suggest Tweaks to a person who is starting to complain of food boredom.

Some tweaking is done earlier on if a person has food intolerances or sensitivities.

The following is a list of Tweaks, grouped by food category. The approximate calorie count is provided in parentheses.

Meats
- Northern Pike - 3.5 oz. (88)
- Catfish - 3.5 oz. (116)
- White Tuna - 3.5 oz. (135)
- Turkey (white meat without skin), roasted - 3.5 oz. (160)
- Pork tenderloin (trimmed of fat) - 3.5 oz. (162)

Meat alternatives
- Egg white - 1 average sized egg (18)
- Egg Beaters - 1/4 cup (30)
- Tofu firm - 3.5 oz. (138)

(NOTE: The OWL Diet is very difficult for vegetarians, so for that reason I do not normally recommend it to vegetarians or vegans).

Vegetables
- Beets - 1/2 cup sliced (37)
- Clausen Sauerkraut - 1/4 cup (5)
- Turnips, raw - 1/2 cup cubed (25)
- Rhubarb, raw - 1/2 cup (13)

Fruits
- Apricot - 1 (17)
- Grapes - count of 10 (36)
- Starfruit - 1 (42)
- Blackberries, fresh - 1/3 cup (21)
- Nectarine - 1 (67)
- Peach - 1 (37)
- Asian Pear - 1 (51)
- Sweet cherries, fresh - 10 (49)
- Plum - 1 (36)
- Pomegranate - 1 (104)
- Raspberries - 1 cup (31)

Grain Carbohydrates
- Oyster Cracker - 1 (4)
- Popcorn air popped - 1 cup (31)

These are the only Tweaks that are permitted. If you get too "into" the Tweaks, you could easily go off track.

PART III:

THE ROUTE TO SUCESS

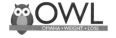

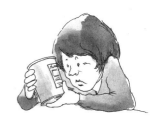

Chapter 9
TIPS FOR SUCCESS

I want you to succeed on the OWL Diet. Since I've "been there, done that" myself, and with hundreds of patients, I have discovered tips to help you stay on track towards achieving permanent weight loss.

I hope you will find the following tips helpful.

1. **Become a very attentive label reader** - Food labels can be deceptive in terms of portion sizes and content, so explore them carefully. Remember that "fat-free" and "sugar free" are usually not calorie free. Even sugar free gum has calories (typically 2-5 calories per piece).

2. **Mustard can be the spice of life** - As you know, ketchup is not permitted on the OWL Diet because it contains a great deal of sugar. Traditional mustard is zero calorie and may be used creatively in sauces and even dressings. Gourmet mustards are typically high in calories and must be avoided. Shop around and you will likely find flavored mustards that are calorie free.

3. **Pickles, too** - Kosher dill pickles (slices or spears), are very low in calories and are permitted in moderation. I have also found sweet pickles, such as gherkins, that are sweetened with Splenda and are therefore lower in calories. Pickled peppers such as yellow banana, cherry or jalapeno are low in calories and make great snacks.

4. **Easy salsa** - If you want salsa, I suggest that you make your own. Dice up some tomatoes and onions, add fresh lemon and lime, and season with cilantro. If you like hot sauces, check the label and you will find that most of them, such as Tabasco, are calorie free.

5. **Seasonings and marinades** - Add seasonings and herbs to your meats, salads and vegetables. Creativity with seasoning adds variety to an otherwise limited selection of foods. Consider marinating your

meats with wine (red with beef, white with chicken, fish or shrimp). Also try using wine or broth when stir frying.

6. **Ceviche with seafood** - Try ceviche, which is fresh fish or shrimp marinated in fresh lime or lemon juice. The acid in the juice softens the proteins in the seafood, and makes it a tender juicy treat. Serve ceviche with fresh onions, tomatoes and cucumbers. Season with fresh herbs.

7. **Easy chicken recipe** - White chicken is a very versatile food with the OWL Diet. Try cooking it in the oven by aligning chicken tenders on a cookie tray, season with herbs and lemon, then cover with a sheet of foil to keep the meat moist. Cook at 350 degrees for 45 minutes, or until tender.

8. **Calorie free soy sauce** – Make Bragg's Liquid Aminos your soy sauce now, and in the future. It may be used in cooking, stir-frying and added to vegetables. Another flavoring option is Worcestershire sauce.

9. **Soups for success** – If you want soup, then you will need to make your own. Purchase a fat free beef or chicken stock (Emeril's brand is one example). You may be surprised to find that beef stock is lower in calories than chicken – opposite to the message about fresh meat. Chicken broth is 10 calories per cup and the beef broth is 5 calories per cup. Add approved vegetables such as tomatoes, onions, celery, chopped spinach and broccoli. Combine the vegetables and broth with diced pieces of chicken or lean beef. Season with salt, pepper, garlic, fresh herbs – and enjoy!

10. **Vinegars** - Most vinegars are either low calorie or zero calorie. After reading the labels, chose vinegars that you can use in cooking or add to a fresh salad. Look for a prepared salad dressing that uses fat free balsamic vinegar (Maple Grove Farms of Vermont has an excellent one).

11. **Zero-calorie brands** - Currently in the United States, we have access to zero-calorie products sold under the brand name Walden Farms. They are available in many grocery stores, or you may order online at: www.waldenfarms.com. Choose from a variety of salad dressings, dips, grilling sauces and toppings that are permitted, as the entire product line is rated as calorie free. When you try these products, please remember that because they are calorie free, they will not taste the same as products packed with fat calories. Walden Farms products do however offer flavor variety that will help you to stay focused and committed to the OWL Diet.

12. **Grain carbohydrates and snacks** - I have found that the OWL Diet grain carbohydrates, such as Melba toast and Italian grissini breadsticks, are best used between meals as snacks or emergency food. If a brief bout of hunger or stomach growling occurs, this is a great food to have on hand. These carbohydrates travel well in the car and on airplanes, and easily fit into a purse or jacket pocket.

13. **Restaurant meals** - The OWL Diet becomes difficult if you are dining out. It is best to avoid the temptations that eating out will offer. If you must eat out, carry your own salad dressing. Order a green salad and perhaps a grilled chicken breast or grilled fish. Specify that you do not want sauce. If the portion is too large, ask your food server to box up the difference, and enjoy it the next day.

14. **Artificial sweeteners** - Any zero-calorie sweetener may be used. Use them to sweeten tea, coffee and as an addition to your fruit. Consider making lemonade using artificial sweeteners. There are also zero-calorie products that may be added to coffee or tea that provide flavors such as mocha and caramel (Splenda makes a good one). Adding cinnamon to coffee after grinding, but before brewing, creates another flavor option.

15. **Sauces** - Try making your own tomato or chili sauces that may be eaten on their own or combined with chicken or beef. For example, combine diced tomatoes, onions, peppers and mushrooms then simmer. The tomatoes will provide the sauce, but you may also add some fat free beef broth or wine. Season and enjoy!

16. **Breading** - For a breading, consider grinding up your allowance of Melba Toast, Ak-Mak crackers or breadsticks and use on chicken, fish or shrimp. Your grain carbohydrates can also be crumbled into salads as croutons.

17. **Creative salads** - Consider adding approved fruits to your salad for a different taste. Apples go very well with romaine and oranges with spinach.

18. **Lettuce wraps** - Wrapping vegetables and meat into a large leaf of romaine with some allowable salad dressing makes a satisfying "sandwich."

19. **Squash for "Pasta"** - Use spaghetti squash tossed with other vegetables or even your own tomato-based sauce and spices for a completely legal "pasta" dish.

The more creative you can be with the foods that are permitted, the more successful you will be on this program.

Be wary of recipes available on the Internet that claim to be approved for use with "HCG Diets." If the ingredients do not fall in line with the approved OWL Diet food list, then they are not to be used.

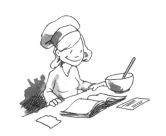

Chapter 10
RECIPES

This chapter contains a series of exceptional recipes, created using Owl Diet approved foods (and the occasional "Tweak").

These recipes were submitted by several of my OWL Diet patients, including Rita Shadden, whose OWL Diet success story is remarkable. Her dedication to losing weight is matched by her commitment to creating these helpful recipes. I owe her a debt of gratitude for her contribution.

My hope is that these recipes will spark your own creativity with OWL Diet Foods. I encourage you to share your ideas for food preparation by submitting your suggestions to: omahamedspa@gmail.com or carterabbott@aol.com.

BREAKFAST

Breakfast is a challenge on the OWL Diet, since dairy products are not allowed. After you reach your target weight, you may go back to enjoying low fat or fat free forms of milk, cheese and yogurt.

Most OWL Dieters start the day with fruit, grain carbohydrates and approved beverages. An example would be: 1 cup of cantaloupe (1/2 of a fruit serving); 2 pieces of Melba Toast with 1 Tbsp. of sugar free Smuckers jam, 12 oz. of water and black coffee with Splenda.

The muffins recipe is delicious and may be incorporated after one month on the OWL Diet (since it contains egg substitute, a "Tweak" food). You can also concoct an omelet using egg substitute and approved vegetables such as mushrooms, tomatoes, peppers and onions.

HIGH FIBER LOW-CALORIE MUFFINS

Total Time	Prep. Time: 20 minutes	Cook Time: 25 minutes
45 minutes	Servings: 12	Yields: 2.2 oz. servings

Ingredients

2 apples, chopped
3/4 cup egg substitute
1/2 cup water
1/2 tsp. cinnamon
1 tsp. vanilla
1 tsp. nutmeg

1 tsp. baking soda
1 tsp. baking powder
2 cups wheat bran
2 tsp. Sweet and Low
1/2 tsp. almond extract
PAM

Directions

- Preheat oven to 400 degrees.
- Blend apples with skin, egg substitute, water, vanilla and almond extract in a blender. Add to dry ingredients and put in a muffin pan sprayed with PAM. Let cool before trying to remove from pan.
- Wrap individually and freeze.

Nutrition Facts

Nutrition information calculated from recipe ingredients.

Amount Per Serving	
Calories 47.14	
Calories from Fat (15%) 7.23	
	% Daily Value
Total Fat 0.8g	1%
Saturated Fat 0.16g	<1%
Cholesterol 13.22mg	4%
Sodium 152.04mg	6%
Potassium 244.08mg	7%
Total Carbohydrates 7.26g	2%
Fiber 5g	20%
Sugar 7.07g	
Protein 0.85g	2%

BALSAMIC MUSHROOMS

Total Time	Prep. Time: 5 minutes	Cook Time: 15 minutes
20 minutes	Servings: 2	Yields: 4.9 oz. servings

Ingredients

8 oz. mushrooms

1 Tbsp. balsamic vinegar

2 sprays PAM

2 Tbsp. water

1 clove garlic, minced

Directions

- Clean mushrooms and cut each in half. Pre-heat a medium size non-stick skillet over medium heat for 3-5 minutes
- Spray the pan with PAM
- Add mushrooms and sauté for 3-5 minutes or until the mushrooms begin to brown. Add balsamic vinegar, minced garlic clove and 1-2 Tbsp. water. Cover and continue cooking 3-5 minutes or until sauce has almost evaporated.
- The mushrooms are ready when the liquid has evaporated leaving only a glaze of balsamic vinegar on them.

Tips

Makes an excellent side dish for baked chicken breast.

Nutrition Facts	Amount Per Serving	
Nutrition information calculated from recipe ingredients.	Calories 29.57	
	Calories from Fat (15%) 4.3	
		% Daily Value
	Total Fat 0.51g	<1%
	Saturated Fat 0.07g	<1%
	Cholesterol 0mg	0%
	Sodium 11.99mg	<1%
	Potassium 393.72mg	11%
	Total Carbohydrates 4.73g	2%
	Fiber 1.17g	5%
	Sugar 2.37g	
	Protein 3.6g	7%

BRAISED CELERY & MUSHROOMS

Total Time	Prep. Time: 15 minutes	Cook Time: 20 minutes
35 minutes	Servings: 2	Yields: 10.4 oz. servings

Ingredients

2 cups celery, sliced diagonally
3/4 cup mushrooms, sliced
1/4 cup onion, chopped

1 chicken bouillon cube
1 cup boiling water
1 tsp. Worcestershire sauce

Directions

- Clean and prepare all vegetables. Place celery in large skillet. Spread mushrooms and onions over the celery.
- Dissolve bouillon in boiling water; add Worcestershire sauce and stir till dissolved. Pour on top of vegetables.
- Bring to a boil, cover, reduce heat, and simmer 10 minutes or until celery is crisp-tender.

Nutrition Facts

Nutrition information calculated from recipe ingredients.

Amount Per Serving	
Calories 42.28	
Calories from Fat (9%) 3.97	
	% Daily Value
Total Fat 0.45g	<1%
Saturated Fat 0.1g	<1%
Cholesterol 0.13mg	<1%
Sodium 370.83mg	15%
Potassium 496.95mg	14%
Total Carbohydrates 8.13g	3%
Fiber 2.52g	10%
Sugar 4.5g	
Protein 2.03g	4%

GRILLED VEGETABLE KABOBS

Total Time	Prep. Time: 15 minutes	Cook Time: 20 minutes
35 minutes	Servings: 4	Yields: 7 oz. servings

Ingredients

1 cup green bell pepper, cut into cubes
1 cup red bell pepper, cut into cubes
1 medium onion, cut in 1" chunks
1/2 lb. mushrooms
1 zucchini, unpeeled and cut in 1/2" slices
4 sprays PAM

Directions

- Clean and cut vegetables into bite size chunks. Thread on skewers. Spray lightly with PAM and cook over grill on low heat until tender crisp, turning frequently.

Tips

If you use wooden skewers, be sure to soak the skewers in warm water 20 minutes before using.

Nutrition Facts

Nutrition information calculated from recipe ingredients.

Amount Per Serving		
Calories 49.91		
Calories from Fat (12%) 5.88		
		% Daily Value
Total Fat 0.68g		1%
Saturated Fat 0.12g		<1%
Cholesterol 0mg		0%
Sodium 11.43mg		<1%
Potassium 473.79mg		14%
Total Carbohydrates 9.62g		3%
Fiber 2.77g		11%
Sugar 4.98g		
Protein 3.26g		7%

ROASTED ASPARAGUS WITH BALSAMIC VINEGAR

Total Time	Prep. Time: 10 minutes	Cook Time: 12 minutes
22 minutes	Servings: 4	Yields: 4.4 oz. servings

Ingredients

40 asparagus spears (small 5" spears)

1/4 tsp. salt

1/4 tsp. fresh ground black pepper

2 tsp. Bragg liquid aminos (i.e. soy sauce)

1 tsp. balsamic vinegar

Lemon zest (optional garnish)

5 sprays butter-flavored cooking spray (i.e. I Can't Believe It's Not Butter)

2 sprays PAM

Directions

- Preheat oven to 400 degrees
- Arrange asparagus in a single layer on a baking sheet coated with PAM. Spray with 2 sprays of spray butter. Sprinkle with salt and black pepper.
- Bake 12 minutes or until tender
- Mix together Bragg liquid aminos and vinegar.
- Drizzle over asparagus, tossing well to coat. Add 3 sprays of I Can't Believe It's Not Butter.

Nutrition Facts	Amount Per Serving	
Nutrition information calculated from recipe ingredients.	**Calories** 25.72	
	Calories from Fat (8%) 2.02	
		% Daily Value
	Total Fat. 0.27g	<1%
	Saturated Fat 0.07g	<1%
	Cholesterol 0mg	0%
	Sodium 308.81mg	13%
	Potassium 248.55mg	7%
	Total Carbohydrates 4.85g	2%
	Fiber 2.55g	10%
	Sugar 2.34g	
	Protein 2.96g	6%

ROASTED ROMA TOMATOES

Total Time 35 minutes	Prep. Time: 5 minutes	Cook Time: 30 minutes
	Servings: 6	Yields: 4.8 oz. servings

Ingredients

6 Roma tomatoes
1 clove garlic, minced
1/2 tsp. sweet basil
1/8 tsp. crushed red pepper flakes

1/8 tsp. salt
1/8 tsp. black pepper
3 sprays PAM

Directions

- Preheat oven to 400 degrees. Line a baking sheet with foil and coat lightly with PAM.
- Combine minced garlic, crushed red pepper, basil, salt and pepper.
- Cut tomatoes lengthwise in half.
- Place tomatoes cut side up on the baking sheet. Sprinkle mixed spices on the tomatoes. Spray with PAM.
- Bake 30-35 minutes, or until they are sizzling and slightly charred. Serve hot.

Nutrition Facts

Nutrition information calculated from recipe ingredients.

Amount Per Serving	
Calories 41.57	
Calories from Fat (12%) 4.82	
	% Daily Value
Total Fat 0.56g	<1%
Saturated Fat 0.08g	<1%
Cholesterol 0mg	0%
Sodium 59.58mg	2%
Potassium 523.1mg	15%
Total Carbohydrates 8.84g	3%
Fiber 2.68g	11%
Sugar 5.74g	
Protein 1.97g	4%

SAUTEED ZUCCHINI WITH ONIONS & ROSEMARY

Total Time	Prep. Time: 13 minutes	Cook Time: 20 minutes
33 minutes	Servings: 4	Yields: 6.3 oz. servings

Ingredients

3 zucchini, thinly sliced
1 onion, thinly sliced
1 tsp. rosemary

Salt to taste
Black pepper to taste
PAM

Directions

- Prepare zucchini and onions.
- Heat a medium size skillet 2-3 minutes over medium heat.
- Spray skillet with PAM. Add onion, cover and sauté 5-10 minutes or until onion becomes soft. If onion begins to stick to skillet add 1-2 Tbsp. water.
- Add zucchini and rosemary. Continue cooking 10 minutes or until zucchini is soft.

Nutrition Facts

Nutrition information calculated from recipe ingredients.

Amount Per Serving		
Calories 38.52		
Calories from Fat (11%) 4.39		
		% Daily Value
Total Fat 0.52g		<1%
Saturated Fat 0.12g		<1%
Cholesterol 0mg		0%
Sodium 16.21mg		<1%
Potassium 432.63mg		12%
Total Carbohydrates 8.02g		3%
Fiber 2.26g		9%
Sugar 3.84g		
Protein 2.13g		4%

SPICED GREEN BEANS

Total Time	Prep. Time: 10 minutes	Cook Time: 25 minutes
35 minutes	Servings: 2	Yields: 7.5 oz. servings

Ingredients

- 2 cups green beans, raw cut into 1" pieces
- 1/2 cup onion, chopped
- 1/2 cup tomato, diced
- 1 clove garlic, chopped
- 1 tsp. oregano, chopped fresh leaves (or dried)
- 1/2 tsp. sea salt
- 2 Tbsp. lemon juice
- 4 sprays PAM

Directions

- Cook beans in salt water until tender, about 20-30 minutes. Drain and rinse.
- In pan prepared with cooking spray (PAM) sauté onion, garlic and tomatoes until tender.
- Combine all ingredients and heat.
- Drizzle with lemon juice and serve.

Nutrition Facts

Nutrition information calculated from recipe ingredients.

Amount Per Serving	
Calories 76.56	
Calories from Fat (10%) 7.7	
	% Daily Value
Total Fat 0.88g	1%
Saturated Fat 0.16g	<1%
Cholesterol 0mg	0%
Sodium 115.23mg	5%
Potassium 497.76mg	14%
Total Carbohydrates 16.89g	6%
Fiber 5.71g	23%
Sugar 5.56g	
Protein 3.32g	7%

STIR-FRIED CABBAGE

Total Time	Prep. Time: 10 minutes	Cook Time: 5 minutes
15 minutes	Servings: 2	Yields: 6.4 oz. servings

Ingredients

2/3 cup celery, sliced diagonally

2 cups cabbage

1/2 cup bell pepper (red or green), chopped

1/3 cup onion, chopped

1 Tbsp. Bragg liquid aminos (i.e. soy sauce)

Pepper to taste

PAM

Directions

- Heat a skillet or wok prepared over medium heat. Spray with PAM.
- Add celery and cook stirring quickly and frequently for 1 minute.
- Add cabbage, bell peppers, and onion. Continue to stir fry until vegetables are tender crisp, about 2-3 minutes.
- Add Braggs, and black pepper to taste. Cook 1 minute longer.

Nutrition Facts

Nutrition information calculated from recipe ingredients.

Amount Per Serving	
Calories 47.46	
Calories from Fat (5%) 2.15	
	% Daily Value
Total Fat 0.27g	<1%
Saturated Fat 0.07g	<1%
Cholesterol 0mg	0%
Sodium 530.23mg	22%
Potassium 347.81mg	10%
Total Carbohydrates 10.48g	3%
Fiber 3.91g	16%
Sugar 5.68g	
Protein 2.91g	6%

CHICKEN SALAD

Total Time	Prep. Time: 5 minutes	Cook Time: 15 minutes
20 minutes	Servings: 1	Yields: 10.2 serving

Ingredients

    1 (3.5 oz.) chicken breast, cooked and cut into small cubes
    6 strawberries, sliced
    1 cup lettuce or baby spinach leaves, shredded
    3 Tbsp. apple cider vinegar
    1 pkg. Sweet and Low or Truvia sweetener
    Salt to taste
    Pepper to taste

Directions

   • Top lettuce or spinach with chicken and strawberries.
   • Mix dressing ingredients together. Sprinkle salad with vinaigrette dressing.

Nutrition Facts

Nutrition information calculated from recipe ingredients.

Amount Per Serving	
Calories 208.27	
Calories from Fat (17%) 34.87	
	% Daily Value
Total Fat 3.89g	6%
Saturated Fat 1.03g	5%
Cholesterol 84.34mg	28%
Sodium 374.62mg	16%
Potassium 508.46mg	15%
Total Carbohydrates 8.6g	3%
Fiber 2.52g	10%
Sugar 5.12g	
Protein 32g	64%

CONFETTI COLESLAW

Total Time	Prep. Time: 15 minutes	Cook Time:
15 minutes	Servings: 4	Yields: 5.2 oz. servings

Ingredients

2 cups red cabbage, thinly shredded
2 cups green cabbage, thinly shredded
1 cup red bell pepper, thinly sliced
1 cup yellow bell pepper, thinly sliced
2 tsp. fresh chives, chopped (optional garnish)
3 Tbsp. apple cider vinegar
1 pinch salt to taste
1 pinch black pepper to taste
2 packets Truvia sweetener (more or less to taste)

Directions

- Wash and prepare all vegetables for the coleslaw.
- Whisk together vinegar and Truvia sweetener to create the dressing for the prepared vegetables. Pour dressing over coleslaw.
- Salt and pepper to taste. Add chives if desired. Marinate in refrigerator 1-2 hours before serving. Toss again before serving.

Tips

This keeps well and is a great side dish for chicken or fish.

Nutrition Facts

Nutrition information calculated from recipe ingredients.

Amount Per Serving	
Calories 39.07	
Calories from Fat (5%) 1.77	
	% Daily Value
Total Fat 0.23g	<1%
Saturated Fat 0.04g	<1%
Cholesterol 0mg	0%
Sodium 91.12mg	4%
Potassium 258.33mg	7%
Total Carbohydrates 9.58g	3%
Fiber 3.21g	13%
Sugar 4.83g	
Protein 1.61g	3%

BEEF & CABBAGE SOUP

Total Time	Prep. Time: 20 minutes	Cook Time: 210 minutes
3 hours 50 minutes	Servings: 10	Yields: 10.5 oz. servings

Ingredients

1 lb. beef top round roast, trimmed of all visible fat and cut into 1/2" cubes

1 onion, chopped	1/4 tsp. dried thyme leaves
2 stalks celery, chopped	1/2 tsp. caraway seeds
1 bell pepper, chopped	9 cups low sodium, fat-free beef
1/2 cup red wine	broth
2 Tbsp. Worcestershire sauce	1/2 head green cabbage, diced
1-1/2 tsp. salt	3 oz. red peppers, roasted and
1/2 tsp. black pepper	drained
1 clove garlic, crushed	2 sprays PAM
1/4 tsp. dried oregano leaves	

Directions

- In a large (6 qt.) pot, sprayed with PAM, add beef. Cook over medium heat, stirring occasionally, until beef is brown. Drain any visible fat. Remove beef from pan.
- Sauté onions, celery, and green peppers in same pan about 4 minutes or until soft and fragrant. Add beef, raise heat to medium high and sauté meat about 3 minutes or until just beginning to take on color.
- Stir in wine, Worcestershire sauce, salt, pepper, garlic, oregano, thyme, and caraway seeds. Stir about 1 minute. Pour in 8 cups broth.
- Add cabbage and red peppers; bring to a boil. Reduce heat and simmer. Partially cover and continue to simmer 3 hours, stirring occasionally. Taste for seasonings and if too thick, add more beef broth.

Nutrition Facts

Nutrition information calculated from recipe ingredients.

Amount Per Serving		
Calories 94.84		
Calories from Fat (26%) 25.08		
		% Daily Value
Total Fat 2.78g		4%
Saturated Fat 0.97g		5%
Cholesterol 29.33mg		10%
Sodium 917.11mg		38%
Potassium 203.72mg		6%
Total Carbohydrates 3.87g		1%
Fiber 0.9g		4%
Sugar 1.75g		
Protein 10.72g		21%

CURRY CAULIFLOWER SOUP

Total Time	Prep. Time: 15 minutes	Cook Time: 35 minutes
1 hour	Servings: 12	Yields: 10.1 oz. servings

Ingredients

2 stalks celery, chopped
1 onion, diced
1/2 cup water
2 tomatoes, peeled, seeded and diced
1 Tbsp. garlic, minced
4 tsp. curry powder (Madras style)

6 cups low sodium, fat-free chicken broth
1 head cauliflower florets
5 sprays PAM
3 scallions, sliced thinly crosswise (optional garnish)

Directions

- Spray a heavy pot with PAM. Combine celery and onions, cover and cook 10 minutes or until tender, stirring occasionally. You may need to add 1/2 cup water to help wilt the onions and celery. Add garlic and cook 5 minutes.
- Stir in the curry powder and cook, stirring, over low heat for 1 minute. Add the broth, cauliflower and tomato. Cook over medium heat till boiling, then simmer for 20 minutes or until the vegetables are very tender.
- Remove the pot from the heat and cool slightly. Puree the soup with a hand held food processer. Season with salt and pepper if desired.

Tips

- Soup may be served HOT or COLD!
- Cooking the curry powder over low heat for a short time eliminates any raw taste and sweetens the spice.

Nutrition Facts

Nutrition information calculated from recipe ingredients.

Amount Per Serving	
Calories 50.47	
Calories from Fat (10%) 5.14	
	% Daily Value
Total Fat 0.6g	<1%
Saturated Fat 0.1g	<1%
Cholesterol 0mg	0%
Sodium 331.48mg	14%
Potassium 560.23mg	16%
Total Carbohydrates 10.78g	4%
Fiber 4.37g	17%
Sugar 4.14g	
Protein 3.65g	7%

FRENCH ONION SOUP

Total Time	Prep. Time: 2 minutes	Cook Time: 10 minutes
12 minutes	Servings: 2	Yields: 6.2 oz. servings

Ingredients

1 cup low sodium, fat-free beef broth

1 med. onion, thinly sliced

1 pinch black pepper to taste

1 dash Worcestershire sauce to taste

3 sprays PAM

Directions

- Sauté onion in pan sprayed with PAM spray until tender and slightly browned. Add beef broth and bring to a boil. Turn down heat. Add Worcestershire sauce and black pepper.
- Turn down heat and simmer 5 minutes.

Nutrition Facts

Nutrition information calculated from recipe ingredients.

Amount Per Serving	
Calories 31.73	
Calories from Fat (12%) 3.81	
	% Daily Value
Total Fat 0.43g	<1%
Saturated Fat 0.08g	<1%
Cholesterol 0mg	0%
Sodium 290.34mg	12%
Potassium 96.28mg	3%
Total Carbohydrates 6.11g	2%
Fiber 1.15g	5%
Sugar 2.62g	
Protein 1.22g	2%

SPICY CURRY WINTER SQUASH SOUP

Total Time	Prep. Time: 20 minutes	Cook Time: 75 minutes
1 hour 35 minutes	Servings: 10	Yields: 8.5 oz. servings

Ingredients

1.5 lb. sbutternut squash, halved

1 lg. onion, peeled and chopped

3 stalks, celery chopped

4 cloves garlic, chopped

1 Tbsp. curry powder (Madras style)

6 cups low sodium, fat-free chicken broth

1/2 tsp. dried oregano leaves

1/2 tsp. dried sage leaves

1/2 Tbsp. hot pepper sauce

Salt to taste

Pepper to taste

PAM

Fresh chives, chopped (optional garnish)

Directions

- Bake squash at 350 degrees for 45 minutes. Scoop out squash. One large squash should yield about 1-1/2 pounds of cooked squash.
- Heat a soup pot over medium-low heat. Spray with PAM, and add the onion and celery and cover. Cook, stirring occasionally, until the onion is translucent, about 8-10 minutes. You may add 1/4 cup water to help the vegetables steam. Add the garlic and cook for 1 minute.
- Add the curry powder, oregano, and sage to the onion mixture and stir till fragrant, about 1 minute. Stir in the squash and then the broth. Bring to a boil over high heat. Reduce the heat to low. Simmer, partially covered, for about 15 minutes. Remove from heat.
- Use a hand held blender to blend the soup to a chunky puree. Season to taste with the hot sauce, salt and pepper. Reheat and serve hot!

Nutrition Facts

Nutrition information calculated from recipe ingredients.

Amount Per Serving	
Calories 46.24	
Calories from Fat (6%) 2.84	
	% Daily Value
Total Fat 0.33g	<1%
Saturated Fat 0.06g	<1%
Cholesterol 0mg	0%
Sodium 391.96mg	16%
Potassium 361.67mg	10%
Total Carbohydrates 11.61g	4%
Fiber 2.08g	8%
Sugar 2.3g	
Protein 1.69g	3%

VEGETABLE SOUP

Total Time	Prep. Time: 10 minutes	Cook Time: 24 minutes
34 minutes	Servings: 5	Yields: 9 oz. servings

Ingredients

- 1/2 cup onion, diced
- 2 cloves garlic, minced
- 3 cups low sodium, fat-free beef broth
- 1-1/2 cups cabbage, diced
- 1 cup raw green beans, cut into 1" pieces
- 1 tomato, diced
- 1 tsp. dried basil leaves
- 1/2 tsp. oregano leaves, crushed
- 1/4 tsp. salt
- 1 cup zucchini, diced
- 2 sprays PAM

Directions

- In a large saucepan, sprayed with PAM, saute the onion and garlic over low heat until softened, about 5 minutes. Add broth, cabbage, beans, tomato, basil, oregano, and salt; bring to a boil. Lower heat and simmer, covered, about 15 minutes or until beans are tender.
- Stir in zucchini and heat 3-4 minutes.

Tips

Chicken or vegetable broth can be substituted for the beef broth.

Nutrition Facts

Nutrition information calculated from recipe ingredients.

Amount Per Serving	
Calories 38.61	
Calories from Fat (7%) 2.81	
	% Daily Value
Total Fat 0.33g	<1%
Saturated Fat 0.06g	<1%
Cholesterol 0mg	0%
Sodium 470.09mg	20%
Potassium 299.96mg	9%
Total Carbohydrates 7.84g	3%
Fiber 2.69g	11%
Sugar 3.44g	
Protein 2.34g	5%

BAKED FISH WITH ITALIAN CRUMB TOPPING

Total Time	Prep. Time: 15 minutes	Cook Time: 10 minutes
25 minutes	Servings: 4	Yields: 4.4 oz. servings

Ingredients

1/4 cup Alessi breadsticks (made from 2 breadsticks crushed)
1/2 tsp. Italian seasoning
1/8 tsp. garlic powder
1/8 tsp. black pepper
1 lb. pollock fish (Any type of white fish may be used for this recipe. The nutritional value for this recipe is based on pollock.)
4 sprays PAM
4 sprays butter-flavored cooking spray (i.e. I Can't Believe It's Not Butter)
1 Tbsp. lemon juice, freshly squeezed
1/2 lemon cut into 4 slices

Directions

- Preheat oven to 450 degrees.
- In a small bowl, stir together the crushed breadsticks, Italian seasoning, garlic powder and pepper; set aside.
- Coat a baking pan with PAM. Place the pollock in the pan, folding under any thin edges of the filets.
- Drizzle filets with the lemon juice, then spoon the crumb mixture evenly on the top. Spray the top of the filets with spray butter.
- Bake in a preheated oven for 10-12 minutes or until the fish flakes easily when tested with a fork and is opaque. Serve with lemon slices.

Nutrition Facts

Nutrition information calculated from recipe ingredients.

Amount Per Serving	
Calories 151.94	
Calories from Fat (15%) 22.2	
	% Daily Value
Total Fat 2.47g	4%
Saturated Fat 0.31g	2%
Cholesterol 103.19mg	37%
Sodium 138.29mg	6%
Potassium 528.51mg	15%
Total Carbohydrates 2.32g	<1%
Fiber 0.35g	1%
Sugar 0.18g	
Protein 28.6g	57%

FOIL BAKED FISH

Total Time	Prep. Time: 5 minutes	Cook Time: 25 minutes
30 minutes	Servings: 1	Yields: 6.1 oz. serving

Ingredients

- 1 4 oz. finfish, cod (Any type of white fish may be used for this recipe. The nutritional value for this recipe is based on cod.)
- 2 oz. lemon juice, freshly squeezed
- 1/4 tsp. salt
- 1/8 tsp. black pepper
- 1/2 tsp. dill weed

Directions

- Preheat oven to 350 degrees
- Place fish on a foil sheet and sprinkle fish with lemon juice, salt, pepper, and dill weed. Wrap tightly with the foil and bake at 350 degrees for 20-25 minutes.

Nutrition Facts

Nutrition information calculated from recipe ingredients.

Amount Per Serving	
Calories 135.18	
Calories from Fat (7%) 9.03	
	% Daily Value
Total Fat 1.01g	2%
Saturated Fat 0.19g	<1%
Cholesterol 62.37mg	21%
Sodium 671.54mg	28%
Potassium 366.97mg	10%
Total Carbohydrates 5.34g	2%
Fiber 0.36g	1%
Sugar 1.36g	
Protein 26.23g	52%

GRILLED SHRIMP WITH CITRUS AND CILANTRO

Total Time	Prep. Time: 40 minutes	Cook Time: 4 minutes
54 minutes	Servings: 4	Yields: 6.6 oz. servings

Ingredients

1 lb. shelled and deveined shrimp or e-z peel shrimp with shell on
2 Tbsp. lemon juice
2 Tbsp. lime juice
1/4 tsp. ground cinnamon
1/4 tsp. paprika
2 Tbsp. fresh cilantro sprigs, chopped
1 clove garlic, minced
Wooden skewers (soaked in water about 30 minutes)
Fresh lemon wedges
PAM

Directions

- Heat grill to high heat. Combine all ingredients and marinate shrimp for about 10 minutes. Do not over marinate.
- Place shrimp on wooden skewers. Spray shrimp with PAM before placing on grill. Grill until shrimp turns pink, about 2 minutes per side. Serve with lemon slices

Tips

Makes an excellent side dish for baked chicken breast.

Nutrition Facts

Nutrition information calculated from recipe ingredients.

Amount Per Serving	
Calories 137.31	
Calories from Fat (14%) 18.58	
	% Daily Value
Total Fat 2.16g	3%
Saturated Fat 0.04g	2%
Cholesterol 172.37mg	57%
Sodium 171.17mg	7%
Potassium 325.56mg	9%
Total Carbohydrates 8.67g	3%
Fiber 2.82g	11%
Sugar 0.34g	
Protein 23.86g	48%

GRILLED SOY BARBECUED SHRIMP

Total Time	Prep. Time: 20 minutes	Cook Time: 8 minutes
58 minutes	Servings: 8	Yields: 4.9 oz. servings

Ingredients

2 lbs. shrimp, raw large
2 cloves garlic, minced
1/2 tsp. sea salt
1/2 cup Bragg liquid aminos (i.e. soy sauce)
1/2 cup lemon juice
3 Tbsp. fresh parsley, finely chopped
2 tsp. onion flakes (dehydrated)
1/2 tsp. black pepper, freshly ground
4 sprays PAM

Directions

- Thaw shrimp if frozen. Shell and devein shrimp leaving tails on.
- Arrange shrimp in shallow glass pan. In small bowl, mash garlic and salt. Stir in remaining ingredients. Pour marinade over shrimp and refrigerate 30 minutes.
- Thread shrimp on skewers. Spray with PAM. Grill approximately 3 minutes basting with the marinade. Turn and grill 3-5 more minutes basting several times.

Nutrition Facts

Nutrition information calculated from recipe ingredients.

Amount Per Serving		
Calories 128.7		
Calories from Fat (14%) 17.9		
		% Daily Value
Total Fat 2.1g		3%
Saturated Fat 0.39g		2%
Cholesterol 172.37mg		57%
Sodium 1155.15mg		48%
Potassium 248.01mg		7%
Total Carbohydrates 3.16g		1%
Fiber 0.2g		<1%
Sugar 0.54g		
Protein 25.09g		50%

ORANGE ROUGHY WITH LEMON, CAPERS & WINE

Total Time	Prep. Time: 5 minutes	Cook Time: 12 minutes
17 minutes	Servings: 2	Yields: 5.6 oz. servings

Ingredients

2 (3 oz.) orange roughy fillets or other delicate white fish fillets
   (Any type of white fish may be used for this recipe.
   The nutritional value for this recipe is based on orange fillets.)
1/2 cup wine
1/2 lemon, thinly sliced
2 tsp. capers, drained
3 Tbsp. water (if needed)
Lemon slice, to decorate

Directions

- Heat a non-stick medium-size skillet over medium-high heat for 3-5 minutes. Add wine. Wine should start to boil as soon as it hits the pan
- Add lemon slices and allow lemon slices to cook with wine over medium heat for 1-2 minutes. Lemons should begin to soften. Add capers.
- Add fish fillets and cook approx. 4 minutes per side
- Be sure sauce does not completely evaporate. You may need to add water to the sauce. You should end up with about 2 tablespoons of sauce when fish is done. Serve fillet with sauce, lemons, and capers poured equally over each fillet. Serve with lemon wedges.

Nutrition Facts

Nutrition information calculated from recipe ingredients.

Amount Per Serving	
Calories 83.67	
Calories from Fat (3%) 2.7	
	% Daily Value
Total Fat 0.39g	<1%
Saturated Fat 0.02g	<1%
Cholesterol 25.5mg	9%
Sodium 1915.21mg	80%
Potassium 157.04mg	4%
Total Carbohydrates 4.9g	2%
Fiber 1.59g	6%
Sugar 0.69g	
Protein 7.38g	15%

SESAME WHITEFISH

Total Time	Prep. Time: 15 minutes	Cook Time: 2 hours
2 hours 25 minutes	Servings: 6	Yields: 5.2 oz. servings

Ingredients

- 1.5 lbs. (4 oz. ea.) finfish, cod (Any type of white fish may be used for this recipe. The nutritional value for this recipe is based on cod.)
- 1/4 cup Rhinegeld German mustard
- 2 Tbsp. Bragg liquid aminos (i.e. soy sauce)
- 4 oz. .dry white wine
- 2 Tbsp. sesame seeds, toasted

Directions

- Place fillets in shallow dish. Mix together mustard, liquid aminos, and wine. Pour evenly over fish. Marinate, covered with plastic wrap, for 1-2 hours in the refrigerator.
- When ready to cook, prepare charcoal grill or preheat oven to a broil.
- Remove fish from marinade and discard marinade. Place fillets on a foil-covered hot grill or broiler pan about four inches from heat or coals, with grill covered. Top with sesame seeds. Cook for approximately 10 minutes or until fish flakes easily, turning once during cooking.

Nutrition Facts

Nutrition information calculated from recipe ingredients.

Amount Per Serving	
Calories 152.39	
Calories from Fat (14%) 20.92	
	% Daily Value
Total Fat 2.47g	4%
Saturated Fat 0.4g	2%
Cholesterol 62.37mg	21%
Sodium 519.83mg	22%
Potassium 304.7mg	9%
Total Carbohydrates 1.21g	<1%
Fiber 0.35g	1%
Sugar 0.2g	
Protein 27.05g	54%

STIR-FRIED GARLIC SHRIMP

Total Time	Prep. Time: 15 minutes	Cook Time: 10 minutes
25 minutes	Servings: 4	Yields: 7.8 oz. servings

Ingredients
- 1 lb. raw shrimp, peeled and deveined
- 2 cloves garlic, finely chopped
- 3 cups mushrooms, sliced
- 1 cup green onions (scallions), sliced into 1" pieces
- 4 oz. dry white wine
- 2 sprays PAM

Directions
- Spray pan with PAM and heat over medium heat.
- Cook and stir garlic for 1 minute. Add shrimp and stir-fry for 2 minutes.
- Stir in mushrooms, green onions, and wine. Stir-fry until shrimp turns pink and vegetables are hot, about 5-7 minutes longer.

Nutrition Facts

Nutrition information calculated from recipe ingredients.

Amount Per Serving	
Calories 167.37	
Calories from Fat (12%) 20.67	
	% Daily Value
Total Fat 2.31g	4%
Saturated Fat 0.42g	2%
Cholesterol 172.37mg	57%
Sodium 176.28mg	7%
Potassium 472.7mg	14%
Total Carbohydrates 5.88g	2%
Fiber 1.21g	5%
Sugar 1.75g	
Protein 25.23g	50%

WHITE FISH WITH DILL, GREEN ONION & BRAGG SAUCE

Total Time	Prep. Time: 10 minutes	Cook Time: 25 minutes
35 minutes	Servings: 1	Yields: 3.9 oz. serving

Ingredients

- 3 oz. finfish, cod (Any type of white fish may be used for this recipe. The nutritional value for this recipe is based on cod.)
- 3 Tbsp. fresh dill, chopped (or 1 tsp. dried)
- 2 Tbsp. green onion, chopped
- 1 Tbsp. Bragg liquid aminos (i.e. soy sauce)
- 1/2 tsp. Worcestershire sauce
- 1/2 tsp. garlic powder
- 1 spray PAM

Directions

- Preheat oven to 350 degrees. Spray 14" sheet of foil with PAM spray and set fillet on center of sheet
- Sprinkle surface of fillet with dill and scallions.
- In a small bowl mix together remaining ingredients and pour over fillet.
- Fold foil over fillet to enclose, crimping edges to seal.
- Place in oven and bake 20-25 minutes or until fish flakes easily with fork.
- Carefully unwrap foil and serve.

Nutrition Facts

Nutrition information calculated from recipe ingredients.

Amount Per Serving		
Calories 102.36		
Calories from Fat (8%) 8.43		
		% Daily Value
Total Fat 1.01g		2%
Saturated Fat 0.18g		<1%
Cholesterol 46.78mg		16%
Sodium 1053.7mg		44%
Potassium 280.16mg		8%
Total Carbohydrates 2.49g		<1%
Fiber 0.46g		2%
Sugar 0.87g		
Protein 21.75g		44%

EASY CHICKEN & BROCCOLI

Total Time 40 minutes	Prep. Time: 10 minutes	Cook Time: 30 minutes
	Servings: 1	Yields: 12 oz. serving

Ingredients

1 (3 oz.) chicken breast, boned and skinned
1 cup broccoli florets, cut into 1" pieces
1 clove garlic, minced
1/2 tsp. fresh ginger-root, minced
3/4 cup low sodium, fat-free chicken-broth
1 dash black pepper
1 dash cayenne pepper or red pepper flakes (if desired)
3 sprays PAM

Directions

- Cut chicken breast into 1" strips.
- Prepare pan with PAM spray. Heat over medium heat and add chicken strips turning until lightly browned on all sides. Remove from skillet and set aside.
- To the same skillet re-spray with PAM; add broccoli, garlic, and ginger. Sauté 1 minute. Reduce heat to low.
- Add chicken strips, spices and chicken broth. Cook stirring occasionally 5-10 minutes until liquid reduces by half.

Nutrition Facts

Nutrition information calculated from recipe ingredients.

Amount Per Serving	
Calories 130.41	
Calories from Fat (14%) 18.4	
	% Daily Value
Total Fat 2.07g	3%
Saturated Fat 0.43g	2%
Cholesterol 49.33mg	16%
Sodium 503.22mg	21%
Potassium 533.19mg	15%
Total Carbohydrates 6.74g	2%
Fiber 0.16g	<1%
Sugar 0.07g	
Protein 22.75g	46%

GRILLED LEMON CHICKEN & VEGETABLE SANDWICH

Total Time	Prep. Time: 10 minutes	Cook Time: 50 minutes
1 hour	Servings: 4	Yields: 11.3 oz. servings

Ingredients

4 Arnold 100% whole wheat sandwich thins
12 oz. (3 oz. ea.) chicken breasts, boned and skinned
3 sprays butter-flavored cooking spray (i.e. I Can't Believe It's Not Butter)
2 Tbsp. lemon juice
2 Tbsp. fresh oregano, chopped   1 portobello mushroom, sliced
1 Tbsp. snipped fresh chives   1/2 red bell pepper, halved
Salt to taste   1/2 red onion, halved
Pepper to taste   4 sprays PAM
1 med. zucchini, thinly sliced
    horizontally

Directions

- In a shallow bowl, stir together, lemon juice, oregano, chives, butter, salt and pepper to taste. Add chicken breasts and turn to coat. Marinate in the refrigerator for 30 minutes or up to 8 hours.
- Spray the zucchini, mushroom, bell pepper, and red onion with PAM. Grill over medium heat for 3-5 minutes on each side, until browned. Cut vegetables into smaller pieces for topping the sandwiches.
- Grill marinated chicken breasts over medium heat for 4-5 minutes on each side, until cooked through. Top with grilled vegetables and serve on sandwich rolls.

Nutrition Facts

Nutrition information calculated from recipe ingredients.

Amount Per Serving	
Calories 234.9	
Calories from Fat (10%) 23.73	
	% Daily Value
Total Fat 2.78g	4%
Saturated Fat 0.41g	2%
Cholesterol 49.33mg	16%
Sodium 367.27mg	15%
Potassium 634.05mg	18%
Total Carbohydrates 29.25g	10%
Fiber 7.81g	31%
Sugar 4.67g	
Protein 26.91g	54%

LEMON-OREGANO CHICKEN SKEWERS

Total Time	Prep. Time: 70 minutes	Cook Time: 10 minutes
1 hour 20 minutes	Servings: 4	Yields: 5.3 oz. servings

Ingredients

16 oz. (8 approx.) chicken-tenders
1 clove garlic, crushed
1/2 lemon, freshly squeezed
1 lemon, cut into 8 wedges
1 tsp. oregano leaves, crushed
1/4 tsp. sea salt
1/8 tsp. black pepper
3 sprays PAM
8 wooden skewers (soaked in water about 30 minutes)

Directions

- Squeeze the juice from half a lemon into a zip-top food bag. Add crushed garlic, oregano, salt, and pepper. Add chicken tenders, seal bag, and turn to mix and coat. Marinate a minimum of 15 minutes and up to 1 hour.
- Spray outdoor grill with PAM and heat.
- Thread one chicken tender onto each skewer and then add a lemon wedge. Grill approximately 4 minutes over a medium heat, turn and grill the other side 4 minutes more, or until chicken is lightly charred and cooked through.

Tips

If you have leftovers, the chicken makes a great salad topper.

Nutrition Facts	Amount Per Serving	
Nutrition information calculated from recipe ingredients.	**Calories** 309.78	
	Calories from Fat (53%) 163.34	
		% Daily Value
	Total Fat 18.16g	28%
	Saturated Fat 3.74g	19%
	Cholesterol 46.49mg	15%
	Sodium 538.29mg	22%
	Potassium 301.08mg	9%
	Total Carbohydrates 21.14g	7%
	Fiber 2.74g	11%
	Sugar 0.62g	
	Protein 17.15g	34%

SOUTHWEST SALSA CHICKEN

Total Time	Prep. Time: 10 minutes	Cook Time: 15 minutes
25 minutes	Servings: 1	Yields: 10.1 serving

Ingredients

- 1 (4 oz.) chicken breasts, boned and skinned
- 1/2 cup onion, chopped
- 1/2 cup tomatoes, diced
- 1 pinch salt to taste
- 1 pinch pepper to taste
- 1 pinch Sweet and Low or Truvia sweetener
- 2 sprays PAM

Directions

- Preheat pan. Spray PAM and sauté all ingredients until fully cooked.

Nutrition Facts

Nutrition information calculated from recipe ingredients.

Amount Per Serving	
Calories 189.66	
Calories from Fat (11%) 20.31	
	% Daily Value
Total Fat 2.27g	3%
Saturated Fat 0.53g	3%
Cholesterol 65.77mg	22%
Sodium 375.56mg	16%
Potassium 760.13mg	22%
Total Carbohydrates 13.8g	5%
Fiber 3.31g	13%
Sugar 7.21g	
Protein 28.43g	57%

ZUCCHINI & CHICKEN

Total Time	Prep. Time: 10 minutes	Cook Time: 28 minutes
38 minutes	Servings: 3	Yields: 8.4 oz. servings

Ingredients

9 oz. (3 oz. ea.) chicken breasts boned and skinned
1/2 cup onion, chopped
1/4 cup bell pepper, chopped
3/4 cup celery, chopped
1 cup zucchini, chopped
1 tomatoes, peeled, seeded and diced
1/2 tsp. garlic, minced
1/2 tsp. oregano leaves, crushed
1/2 tsp. basil, chopped
1/4 tsp. salt
1/4 tsp. fresh ground black pepper
2 sprays PAM

Directions

- Spray a non-stick skillet with PAM. Brown chicken over medium heat. Add the onion, green pepper, and celery.
- Sauté for 5-8 minutes, adding 1/4 cup of water and covering with a lid to steam the vegetables.
- Turn chicken and add the zucchini and tomato. Add spices and simmer for 20 minutes, stirring once or twice.

Nutrition Facts	Amount Per Serving	
Nutrition information calculated from recipe ingredients.	Calories 134.68	
	Calories from Fat (10%) 13.98	
		% Daily Value
	Total Fat 1.57g	2%
	Saturated Fat 0.38g	2%
	Cholesterol 49.33mg	16%
	Sodium 282.54mg	12%
	Potassium 640.05mg	18%
	Total Carbohydrates 8.56g	3%
	Fiber 2.59g	10%
	Sugar 4.64g	
	Protein 21.44g	43%

SWISS STEAK

Total Time	Prep. Time: 15 minutes	Cook Time: 90 minutes
1 hour 45 minutes	Servings: 6	Yields: 4.9 oz. servings

Ingredients
1 lb. beef top round steak, cut 3/4" thick
1 tomato, peeled, seeded and diced
1 onion, thinly sliced
1 bell pepper, thinly sliced
1/2 tsp. salt
1/2 tsp. fresh ground black pepper
3 sprays PAM

Directions
- Spray pan with PAM. Brown the steak on both sides.
- Add vegetables and cover. Simmer about 1 hour and 15 minutes or to desired doneness.

Nutrition Facts

Nutrition information calculated from recipe ingredients.

Amount Per Serving	
Calories 206.91	
Calories from Fat (62%) 128.26	
	% Daily Value
Total Fat 14.24g	22%
Saturated Fat 5.66g	28%
Cholesterol 48.38mg	16%
Sodium 91.89mg	4%
Potassium 378.28mg	11%
Total Carbohydrates 4.36g	1%
Fiber 1.15g	5%
Sugar 2.3g	
Protein 14.94g	30%

BBQ RUB MIX

Total Time	Prep. Time: 5 minutes	Cook Time:
15 minutes	Servings: 30	Yields: 0.1 oz. servings

Ingredients

6 Tbsp. sea salt
4 Tbsp. sweet paprika
2 Tbsp. hot paprika

1 Tbsp. dry mustard
1/2 tsp. cayenne pepper
1/2 tsp. black pepper

Directions

- Mix together all ingredients. Store in a glass jar.
- Sprinkle meat with rub and set in refrigerator to marinate 30 minutes before cooking.

Tips

Stores well for up to six months.

Nutrition Facts

Nutrition information calculated from recipe ingredients.

Amount Per Serving	
Calories 7.24	
Calories from Fat (34%) 2.47	
% Daily Value	
Total Fat 0.28g	<1%
Saturated Fat 0.03g	<1%
Cholesterol 0mg	0%
Sodium 820.7mg	34%
Potassium 34.8mg	<1%
Total Carbohydrates 1.2g	<1%
Fiber 0.59g	2%
Sugar 0.15g	
Protein 0.31g	<1%

BAKED APPLES

Total Time	Prep. Time: 5 minutes	Cook Time: 20 minutes
25 minutes	Servings: 1	Yields: 6 oz. serving

Ingredients
1 apple, cored and sliced into 8 wedges
2 Tbsp. water
1 pkg. Sweet and Low or Truvia sweetener
1/2 tsp. vanilla
1/4 tsp. cinnamon

Directions
- Wash, quarter and remove apple core. Put apple in microwave safe dish with water and vanilla. Sprinkle top of apple with cinnamon and sugar substitute.
- Microwave on high for approximately 3-5 minutes, or bake at 350 degrees for approximately 20 minutes.

Tips
The skins of Delicious apples tend to be tough, so you may want to try other varieties of apples. Peeling the apples will result in a loss of fiber.

Nutrition Facts	Amount Per Serving	
Nutrition information calculated from recipe ingredients.	Calories 79.41	
	Calories from Fat (3%) 2.04	
		% Daily Value
	Total Fat 0.24g	<1%
	Saturated Fat 0.04g	<1%
	Cholesterol 0mg	0%
	Sodium 2.52mg	<1%
	Potassium 153.87mg	4%
	Total Carbohydrates 19.85g	7%
	Fiber 3.66g	15%
	Sugar 14.62g	
	Protein 0.39g	<1%

Chapter 11
VITAMINS AND SUPPLEMENTS

The OWL Diet teaches you to enjoy fresh healthy food. You are eating large quantities of nutrient rich vegetables, adequate amounts of fruit, low fat meats and a very limited amount of grain carbohydrates.

Certain supplements and vitamins are recommended with the OWL Diet to enhance your outcome. These supplements will help maintain bone health, provide energy for daily activities, promote regular bowel movements, and proper muscle function. With a Low Calorie Diet (LCD), acidosis occurs as fat is burned to generate energy, and this may lead to electrolyte imbalance, such as low potassium levels. The OWL Diet stands apart from older versions of the HCG Diet by emphasizing the need for vitamins and other supplements.

When you are buying nutritional supplements, remember that the cheapest is not necessarily the best. Look for good quality products from reputable manufacturers.

CALCIUM WITH VITAMIN D

The OWL Diet does not allow the use of any milk or dairy products. Although you will receive calcium from spinach, broccoli, brussel sprouts and related vegetables, it is still mandatory that you take a calcium and vitamin D supplement. This is very important for maintenance of bone health. The calcium may also alleviate symptoms of increased stomach acidity and acid reflux.

Take 1,000 to 1,500 mg. of calcium carbonate daily and 200 to 800 IU of vitamin D daily. Often they are combined in one product. Tablets that can be swallowed whole, chewed, or liquid forms are all acceptable. The total daily caloric intake of this supplement should be less than 10 calories.

B-COMPLEX VITAMINS

A quality B-complex vitamin is necessary for supporting adequate energy, the immune system, and mood stability. Look for a B-Complex Vitamin that provides the following amounts per day:

- Thiamine 100mg.
- Riboflavin 100mg.
- Niacinamide 100mg.
- Vitamin B-6 (Pyridoxine) 100mg.

VITAMIN B-12

In addition to the B-complex supplement, I find that extra Vitamin B-12 is helpful to boost energy levels. As we age, our ability to absorb B-12 is often diminished. In addition, surgeries on the stomach and intestine may further inhibit B-12 absorption. Taking supplements of B-12 by mouth may be adequate for some people, but for others a source of sublingual (under the tongue), or B-12 by injection can be very helpful.

Fortunately, B-12 is non-toxic even when taken in high doses, so it is safe for you to self medicate with sublingual or Intramuscular (IM) injections. Sublingual B-12 may be purchased without a prescription at the pharmacy or supplement stores. Choose a form of sublingual that easily dissolves under the tongue.

I prefer having OWL Diet participants use B-12 by IM injection. In the United States, B-12 injections are only available from a doctor or by prescription. The dose of 1,000 mcg. is administered once or twice per week. In the med spa, the injections are given by the doctor, nurse or trained medical assistant.

Patients may also learn to perform B-12 shots at home. B-12 is stored in a dark bottle to protect it from sunlight. It should be stored at room temperature, in a cupboard. We teach patients how to withdraw the sterile liquid B-12 from a bottle and inject it into the thigh muscle in the same fashion as HCG is administered.

MELATONIN

Melatonin is a hormone that is naturally produced by the pineal gland in the brain. As a supplement, it is often used to enhance sleep. We do know that an adequate amount of restful sleep is very important for success in losing weight.

If you need assistance getting to sleep, then supplemental melatonin may be helpful. The dose range that I advise is 2 mg. to 4 mg. in a controlled release tablet, taken one hour before bedtime.

FIBER SUPPLEMENTS

Many people on the OWL Diet find their pattern of bowel movements will often change. Even people with a normal regular pattern of daily or twice daily bowel movements will typically notice a decrease in their bowel habit. Stools are often firmer and harder.

The result can be uncomfortable straining to have a bowel movement, that in turn can lead to anal fissures or hemorrhoids. Constipation may also develop, leading to bloating, abdominal discomfort and back pain.

A weekly OWL Diet visit with less or no weight loss may be a sign of constipation.

I discuss bowel pattern at the initial consultation. If someone has less than one bowel movement per day before starting my diet, then I recommend a fiber supplement. Adequate fluid intake is simply not enough to prevent constipation.

The choice of fiber supplement is important, as it must be very low in calories. One example is sugar free psyllium powder that is mixed with water (Sugar Free Metamucil brand, as an example). The other option is a variety of non-absorbable fiber capsules and tablets. A side effect of fiber supplements may be increased gas production.

If a patient has not had a bowel movement for four days, then it's time for a laxative. That topic is dealt with in Chapter 16.

POTASSIUM

As your body burns off fat for calories, acids are formed. This is essentially a medically managed ketoacidosis. With a drop in pH (acidity level), the body may also experience a drop in potassium levels.

Lower potassium levels may cause muscle weakness or cramping. If this occurs, speak to your doctor about the possibility of adding a potassium supplement. Not all participants are candidates for potassium supplements, based on other medications taken and kidney function.

Potassium is present in oranges, so choosing them as one or both of your fruits may be sufficient. An over-the-counter potassium supplement is typically sold as a 99 mg. tablet, and one or two a day may be needed, but take it only on the advice of your doctor.

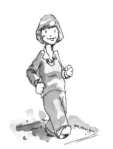

Chapter 12
EXERCISE AND THE OWL DIET

I mentioned exercise and the OWL Diet earlier in this book, but the subject deserves further discussion because it is so important for you to fully understand the role of mild exercise while you are on the diet.

Exercise is a vital component of good health. Regular exercise has been shown to reduce the risk for heart disease, strengthen bones, maintain joint flexibility and manage blood pressure as well as blood sugar (to mention just a few benefits). I'm most certainly a proponent of exercise and lots of it.

With the OWL Diet, we are limiting your caloric intake. The Low Calorie Diet (LCD) does not provide you with the energy that you would need to expend to exercise in a highly active way. You'll have adequate energy to perform day-to-day activities.

When you are on the OWL Diet, I do *not* allow you to exercise to the point that:

- Your heart rate increases to over 120.
- You are breathing hard.
- You are sweating heavily.

Examples of exercise that is *not* permitted include:

- Running
- Walking over 3.5 mph, especially on an incline
- Pushing hard on a bicycle ride
- Swimming more than one length of a full size pool
- Weight lifting over 10 pounds

Keep in mind that most people have activities that are part of their day-to-day routines that qualify as mild to moderate exercise. Examples of these activities include:

- House cleaning
- Yard work
- Mowing the lawn
- Laundry

You should feel fine performing these day-to-day activities, but you may need to undertake them at a slower pace and divide the activities up over several days.

Do not undertake new activities that were not a part of your routines prior to starting the OWL Diet. When in doubt, it is always best to consult your physician.

If during the course of day-to-day activities you feel lightheaded, weak or dizzy, then take a break and consume additional water as well as foods that are

Acceptable Exercises on the OWL Diet:

Examples of light activity that are acceptable (with approval of your physician) are:

- *Leisurely walking outdoors or on a treadmill, on level ground, for 15-30 minutes*
- *Light pool activity including stretching and leisurely swimming*
- *Leisurely riding a bicycle on level ground for 15 minutes*
- *Light yoga for 15-30 minutes*
- *Stretching for muscle tone and flexibility*
- *Use of hand weights of up to 10 pounds for 10 minutes*

approved on the LCD. If you continue to feel unwell, then contact your doctor or seek immediate medical attention.

As I mentioned earlier, patients who insist on continuing strenuous physical activity invariably fail on the OWL Diet because they lack sufficient energy to continue or they find they are unable to control their hunger, even with HCG injections.

When you complete your OWL Diet and you've reached your goal weight, you can engage in more physical activity. In fact, I think you'll find it will be much more enjoyable because of your lower weight.

Regular physical exercise is an excellent way for you to *maintain* the weight you've lost.

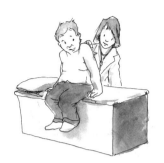

Chapter 13
MEDICAL CONDITIONS AND THE OWL DIET

Many of us have experienced serious medical conditions related to being overweight, such as diabetes, heart disease and high blood pressure. It is not surprising that people with one or more of these serious medical conditions desire to undertake the OWL Diet.

I can happily report that for most of them, the results are positive and not only have they lost weight, they have improved their overall health.

Although my statements here are well supported by current medical knowledge, I have also included my personal observations and opinions as to how the OWL Diet may interact in a positive or negative way with these medical conditions.

Always consult with your personal physician(s) before undertaking a low calorie diet, and the use of prescription medications.

DIABETES MELLITUS

Type 2 diabetes mellitus occurs frequently in overweight patients. A problem we call "insulin resistance" is typically present, whereby the body is producing insulin, but defects occur at the cellular level that interfere with the functions that insulin normally performs.

When an overweight person with Type 2 diabetes loses weight, in most cases blood sugar control will improve, insulin resistance will decrease and the need for medication will lessen.

In some cases, by achieving a normal body weight, some people are able to stop medication altogether.

Over time, many people with Type 2 diabetes also end up taking insulin, which may in turn trigger an undesirable weight gain. Once again, partnership with your physician to carefully monitor medication requirements combined with daily blood sugar measurement is mandatory, while following the OWL Diet.

Type 1 diabetes mellitus is entirely different, and occurs when cells in the pancreas gland that are responsible for producing insulin fail. The result is low to absent levels of naturally produced insulin. Type 1 diabetics are totally dependent on administered insulin.

At the time of diagnosis, most people with Type 1 diabetes are not over-weight, and may in fact have lost weight leading up to their diagnosis. With the institution of prescribed insulin in people with Type 1 diabetes, any weight that was lost is typically recovered, and sometimes additional undesirable weight is gained.

With a healthy diet, and regular activity, most Type 1 diabetics are able to keep their weight at an ideal Body Mass Index (BMI). However, some Type 1 diabetics do become overweight and this can interfere with healthy blood sugar control.

In these circumstances, the Type 1 diabetic can participate in the OWL Diet, but only after careful consultation with the treating physician, regular home blood sugar testing and regular visits with a doctor.

In this scenario, people with diabetes, and the people who live with them, need to know how to recognize the symptoms of low blood sugar (hypoglycemia) and have a clear plan on how to manage blood sugars that are too low.

HYPERTENSION

Elevated blood pressure is called hypertension. Obesity is a major risk factor for developing hypertension. Weight loss can have a profound effect on lowering blood pressure if you already have hypertension. Frequent monitoring of Blood Pressure (BP) is necessary when you participate with the OWL Diet and have hypertension. Medication dose adjustments are common.

In my experience, BP can drop quickly and dramatically in some individuals. If you start developing symptoms of dizziness, lightheadedness or fatigue, then it may be a sign that your blood pressure is too low. Check with your doctor before reducing or stopping any medications.

Other risk factors for developing hypertension include a positive family history of increased BP, smoking, lack of physical activity and excessive sodium chloride (salt) intake. Limit your salt intake on the OWL Diet and consider the use of salt substitutes. Once you achieve your weight loss goal, a regular exercise routine is important.

You may have an ideal body weight, and still have a diagnosis of hypertension, with the need for BP lowering medications.

HYPERLIPIDEMIA

Elevated cholesterol is frequently caused by genetics. A family history of high cholesterol may genetically program you to overproduce cholesterol.

The effect of weight loss on lowering cholesterol is typically favorable, but the overall reduction may be less than anticipated. People with a normal BMI, and low fat diet, may still have elevated cholesterol.

The OWL Diet is very low in fat and oil (virtually none is allowed) and continuation of a low fat diet for life will help maintain your cholesterol at healthier levels.

The other lipid of concern is triglycerides. Elevated triglyceride levels are more closely aligned with obesity, but the condition also has a genetic basis. Weight loss can play a very significant role in lowering triglycerides.

During the OWL program, I typically recommend that you continue any prescribed lipid lowering medications (such as "statins" or "fibrates"). If you have an established diagnosis of coronary artery disease, heart disease, peripheral arterial disease or cerebrovascular disease (such as TIA's or stroke), then your doctor may not want you to stop your prescribed therapies.

Fish oil may be used to assist in lipid control, either in prescription or over-the-counter forms. If you take more than one capsule of fish oil daily, it may be advisable to stop the fish oil, as the oil content may actually interfere with your weight loss. Only stop fish oil after consultation with your doctor.

CORONARY HEART DISEASE

Coronary Heart Disease (CHD) occurs when there are blockages in the arteries that supply oxygen to the heart. Other names for CHD include coronary artery disease and arteriosclerosis. CHD may lead to angina pectoris, heart attack (acute coronary syndrome) and congestive heart failure.

If you have coronary heart disease, your doctor must determine that you are stable before you are a candidate for the OWL Diet.

If there has been any change in your heart condition in the previous six months, I do not advise participation in this program for weight loss.

A diseased heart is often more susceptible to the changes in blood pH (ketoacidosis) and potassium levels that may occur during the course of treatment with HCG and a LCD.

This is one of the reasons that I never endorse the VLCD (Very Low Calorie Diet of 500 calories per day) program. At that level of calorie restriction, there is the potential for unsafe levels of ketoacidosis, that might adversely affect heart function, including the development of arrhythmias that may even be life threatening. Once again the potential risk of a weight loss program needs to be weighed against the risk of remaining obese.

ARTHRITIS

There are many forms of arthritis, but the most common type is called Osteoarthritis (OA) that affects weight-bearing joints, such as the knees and hips.

Risk factors for OA include previous joint injury (trauma), age, family history and obesity. Obesity places added strain on weight-bearing joints.

With successful weight loss on the OWL Diet, many people report a reduction in joint pain. Certainly the control of obesity at any stage in life will have positive effects on joint function and mobility.

SLEEP APNEA

People with sleep apnea experience partial obstruction of the air passage when sleeping, resulting in a combination of snoring, awakening, apnea (pause in breathing) and poor sleep quality. Obesity is one of the risk factors for sleep apnea.

With weight loss, the degree of sleep apnea frequently improves. If you have been prescribed a CPAP machine, then you should keep using it while you are losing weight. After successful weight loss, then consult with your doctor to see if a repeat sleep study is needed to determine if CPAP is still needed. Do not stop CPAP without receiving medical advice first.

INFERTILITY

There are many causes of infertility, but as a general statement it can be said that obesity can affect hormone levels, and in women, this can affect the regularity of the menstrual cycle and fertility.

Polycystic Ovary Syndrome (PCOS) is part of a broader condition recognized as Metabolic Syndrome (formerly Syndrome X), that occurs more commonly in overweight individuals. One feature of this condition is reduced fertility.

Loss of unwanted fat can, in certain cases, improve fertility.

CANCER

Cancer is a very large and diverse topic. Obesity has been established as a risk factor for certain cancers, including breast and endometrial (uterine) cancer. Losing weight will reduce the risk for some individuals.

When a history of cancer already exists, then you need to discuss the OWL Diet openly with your oncologist. You may be advised not to use HCG, even in low doses.

Men with a history of cancer of the prostate or testicular cancer should not participate in the HCG OWL Diet.

GALL BLADDER AND PANCREATIC PROBLEMS

Inflammation of the gall bladder is called cholecystitis. It typically leads to the surgical removal of the gall bladder. Obesity is one of the risk factors for cholecystitis.

Ironically, in the era of bariatric surgery (weight loss surgery), there is also a clear indication that rapid weight loss can trigger a gall bladder problem.

With the OWL Diet, the rate of weight loss is typically slower than that seen with successful bariatric surgery. As a result, my experience has been that development of a gall bladder problem while on the LCD is uncommon.

I always tell my patients that a gall bladder problem may occur at any time in their life, and may therefore occur while they are on any diet.

People with a history of pancreatitis should not participate in the OWL Diet.

IRRITABLE BOWEL SYNDROME

Irritable Bowel Syndrome (IBS) is a very common condition affecting men and women. My observation has been that when people follow the OWL Diet, they are eliminating most processed foods and all dairy products.

The result is that the majority of people with IBS report less bloating, abdominal discomfort and less flatus. Some patients have reported that their IBS has gone away as long as they continue a healthy eating pattern.

Some patients with IBS suffer from severe constipation before starting the OWL Diet. This group desires special consideration. On the OWL Diet, your bowel pattern will typically change to become less frequent with firmer, harder stools. If a person suffers from constipation before the OWL Diet, they require medical advice that might lead to the use of a combination of calorie free fiber supplements, stool softeners and laxatives as needed.

GERD

GERD is short for gastroesophageal reflux disease. In this condition, stomach acid migrates into the esophagus. The human esophagus is not designed to handle the acidity and the presence of acid there causes burning or discomfort. Over time, the acid exposure may result in changes to the lining of the esophagus that may cause narrowing (strictures) or cellular changes (Barrett's) that may in turn lead to esophageal cancer.

Although GERD is caused by several factors, there is no question that abdominal obesity creates a mechanical pressure on the stomach that increases the risk or severity of GERD. As a result, weight loss is often associated with an improvement in this condition, with fewer symptoms and possibly less need for medication to treat GERD.

A group of medications called Proton Pump Inhibitors (including Nexium, Prilosec and Prevacid), reduce stomach acid production, and are often prescribed for GERD. When used daily, these medications have been demonstrated to adversely affect the absorption of vitamin B-12. In these patients, use of supplemental vitamin B-12 by injection once to twice per week is very important while you are on the OWL Diet.

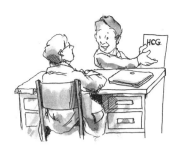

Chapter 14

GETTING YOUR DOCTOR ON BOARD WITH THE OWL DIET

Congratulations on your decision to take control of your weight problem. With the OWL Diet you will quickly and safely lose weight, and learn how to keep it off.

You may be reading this book because you are one of my patients at the Omaha Med Spa in Omaha, Nebraska. I will be your weight loss doctor, and guide you on your journey to permanent weight loss.

If you live outside the Omaha area, you will need to find a doctor to supervise your program. That may be a doctor who has a special interest in weight control or it may be your primary care doctor (family doctor, GP, internist or gynecologist). This chapter is designed to help your doctor understand the OWL Diet, and how he or she can help you achieve your weight loss goal.

Here are some frequently asked questions.

HOW DO I OBTAIN HCG?

Human Chorionic Gonadotropin (HCG) is available in the United States by prescription from a licensed physician. Purchasing HCG without a valid prescription is illegal. That has not stopped inappropriate sale of HCG through the internet. I do not support the sale or purchase of HCG through the internet, without a valid prescription, or the use of HCG for weight loss without medical supervision.

Furthermore, as a consumer you cannot be assured of the quality or authenticity of HCG that you may be purchasing over the internet.

The best solution is to obtain HCG from a physician affiliated with a weight loss facility or medical spa in your community.

The alternative is to ask your primary care physician (often the doctor who knows you best) for a prescription for HCG that can then be filled by a pharmacy. This second option may pose some challenges for the following reasons:

1. Most physicians have either not heard of using HCG to lose weight, or their knowledge of the program is limited.
2. Physicians practice in a conservative, highly regulated environment. They do not always embrace ideas that are considered unconventional.
3. Physicians are taught that weight loss is best achieved by "reduced intake of calories and increased exercise." Low calorie dieting has been inappropriately labeled as being "high risk."
4. Your physician may be concerned about your ability to administer HCG injections at home.

HOW DO I PAY FOR HCG?

The following applies to United States residents as of the writing of this book. For updated IRS regulations, refer to: www.IRS.gov and your accountant for further advice.

As of 2010, some employers permit employees to contribute to Flexible Spending Accounts (FSA), sometimes called "Cafeteria Plans." Also, individuals who hold health insurance plans with a high deductible are able to contribute pre-tax dollars into a Health Savings Account (HSA). Check to see if you can use these funds to help pay for the OWL Diet, which is a medically prescribed program of weight loss.

HOW DO I CONVINCE MY DOCTOR TO PROVIDE A PRESCRIPTION FOR HCG?

I'm including here some powerful arguments in favor of the OWL Diet and the use of HCG. They'll help you assure your doctor that HCG for weight loss is:

1. Safe for you
2. Important for you as a means to take control of your health problems that are aggravated by your current weight
3. Easily performed by injection at home, with the help of this book

Be prepared for your doctor visit.

Do you have one or more of the following medical conditions that are aggravated by obesity?

- Hypertension (high blood pressure)
- Coronary Artery Disease (Angina Pectoris, history of "heart attack")
- Congestive heart failure
- Osteoarthritis
- Chronic back pain
- Diabetes Mellitus Type 2
- Infertility secondary to obesity
- Metabolic Syndrome
- Polycystic Ovary Syndrome
- Hyperlipidemia - high cholesterol or high triglycerides
- Snoring
- Sleep apnea
- Depression aggravated by poor self-image due to obesity
- Family history of breast cancer

If you have any of the above, point out to your doctor that you want to partner with him/her to lose weight and take control of some of your health problems.

1. You will need to point out to your doctor that HCG has been used for decades to assist people to lose weight. Also, explain to your doctor that The OWL Diet, as created by Dr. Carter Abbott, allows 600-700 calories per day and is therefore very safe (as opposed to the original Very Low Calorie Diet of 500 calories per day).
2. Explain that you have an understanding of the physical effects of lower calorie dieting. Tell your doctor that you want to have medical supervision which includes weekly visits to be weighed and monitored for changes in blood pressure and blood sugar (as needed).
3. Your doctor may ask you to have a full physical examination and blood work prior to starting the OWL Diet. This is an ideal situation for you. As part of your working together with your doctor, it

is important to allow him or her to share the medical management of your use of HCG, and the monitoring of the weight loss. In most cases the cost of a full physical exam and blood work will be covered by your insurance company as a preventative care exam.

4. Your doctor will advise you if there is a charge for the weekly visits, or if it will be billed to insurance. Insurance companies do not currently cover the cost of weight loss programs for obesity, but will cover the cost of care for medical conditions affected by obesity such as diabetes mellitus, heart disease and hypertension. Most of the components of the weekly visits may be performed by nurses or medical assistants familiar with the OWL Diet, and under physician supervision.

5. Your doctor may point out that HCG is not FDA approved for weight loss. Although this is correct, you can point out accurately that many FDA approved medications are used for "off label" purposes. This frequently occurs. Examples in the aesthetic world include the use of Botox in areas other than frown lines and Juvederm in areas other than nasolabial folds.

6. Finally, if your doctor is still unsupportive, then offer him or her the "Open Letter to Physicians" written by me, Dr. Abbott, and is shown at the end of this chapter.

7. And as an added level of comfort for your physician, I suggest you show him or her the "Consent for The OWL Diet" form that I have developed and is shown at the end of this chapter.

Simply photocopy these two forms with a copy of the actual OWL Diet and provide them to your physician.

An Open Letter to Physicians

Dear Doctor,

Your patient is offering you this letter because he or she has researched the benefits of weight loss with the OWL Diet that I have developed. OWL stands for "Omaha Weight Loss" and it is the result of working with hundreds of patients to develop a safe and effective way to lose an average of 15 to 20 pounds per month.

Prior to starting an aesthetics practice, I was a primary care physician for 25 years. During that time I found it very difficult to get my patients to lose weight. As part of my conservative training, I advised my overweight patients to "eat less and exercise more." As you may have discovered yourself, the success rate with that approach is very low. Most of my time with obese patients was spent managing the medical problems that obesity had caused, such as hypertension, heart disease, diabetes mellitus and arthritis.

I researched the original HCG Diet and found that there were many myths and inaccuracies. The OWL Diet represents a significant update, incorporating enhanced food selection, a higher calorie allowance of 600-700 calories per day and other modifications that enhance safety while maintaining efficacy. I personally lost 20 pounds in five weeks on the OWL Diet, and it taught me how to eat differently, and maintain the weight loss.

Your patient needs your help in two ways:
1. We need you to write a prescription for HCG, syringes and a sharps disposal container. Here is a sample prescription:

   Rx:

   (1) HCG Injectable

   Pharmacist to reconstitute:

   To a dilution of 125 IU per 0.5cc

   Qty: 15cc in a multidose vial of bacteriostatic water (one month supply)

   Patient Directions:

   Administer 125 IU into the thigh, once daily in the morning for four weeks.

   (2) 3cc Syringe Combination with 25G 5/8" Needle

   Qty: 30

   (3) Sharps Container

   Qty: 1

   It has been my experience that it is very safe and easy to teach most patients how to self-inject HCG into the anterior thigh muscle.

2. Secondly, your patient requires your medical supervision. He or she may benefit from a complete physical examination prior to starting the OWL Diet. In addition, bloodwork may be needed such as CBC, Complete Metabolic Panel, Lipid Panel and a TSH. Your patient knows that you will ultimately decide which blood tests, if any, are needed.

I advise patients on the OWL Diet to be seen weekly to be weighed. In some cases, a blood pressure measurement may be helpful. Additional monitoring will vary depending on the medical conditions that they have (such as home blood glucose monitoring for diabetics).

I encourage you to use the "Consent for The OWL Diet" that I have developed and is attached to this message.

Thank you for your assistance, and for keeping an open mind to this unique and highly effective method of weight loss.

Sincerely,
Carter Abbott, MD
Omaha Med Spa
14450 Eagle Run Drive, Unit #260
Omaha NE, 68116
Phone: 402-614-5556

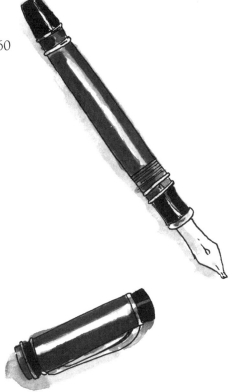

Consent for Omaha Weight Loss (OWL) Diet

Name: _____ DOB: _____

HCG stands for human chorionic gonadotropin. It is produced in large amounts by pregnant women and does not otherwise occur naturally in men or women. Since the 1940s, it has been combined with very low calorie dieting to accomplish weight loss. The benefit of HCG is reported to be a reduced appetite, maintenance of energy and the loss of unwanted fat. The OWL Diet uses a low calorie diet of approximately 600-700 calories per day that results in an average weight loss of 15-20 pounds per month.

There are very few clinical studies on the use of HCG for weight loss. HCG is FDA approved for infertility. Use of HCG for weight loss is considered "Off Label" and is not FDA approved. The FDA states that "HCG has not been demonstrated to be effective adjunctive therapy in the treatment of obesity."

You should *not* use the OWL Diet if you:
- Are pregnant, planning on becoming pregnant during treatment, or are breast feeding
- Have a history of cancer of the prostate or testicular cancer
- Have had a heart attack in the last three months
- Have a history of uncontrolled gout, or heart disease (including undiagnosed chest pain, shortness of breath)
- Have a history of active gallbladder disease or pancreatitis

The *risks* of the OWL Diet include:
- Changes in blood pressure, blood sugar and electrolytes that may cause weakness, fainting or cardiac irregularities
- Less weight loss than you were hoping to achieve
- Mild discomfort, bruising and a low risk of infection from HCG injections
- Flare-up or development of gout or gall bladder problems
- Weight loss may cause temporary loss of menstrual periods, or irregular periods

The **benefits** of weight loss may include:
- An improved sense of confidence, self-esteem and well-being
- Improvement in blood pressure, cholesterol, triglycerides and improvement of abnormal blood sugars
- Improvement of infertility if it is associated with obesity
- Reduced risk for heart disease and many types of cancer
- Reduced joint pain
- Reduction of sleep apnea

By signing this form, I agree to provide a full disclosure of current and past medical problems, and current medications that I take. I also agree to attend all required treatment visits and follow the diet guidelines provided.

By signing this form, I agree that I understand this consent form and all my questions have been answered to my satisfaction.

Patient Signature	*Date*	*Witness Signature*

OWL Diet Progress

Below is a sample of a progress note that may be used by medical offices and patients to track weekly progress.

For each visit C refers to cycle number, and W refers to the week of the OWL Diet just completed. For example: **C** 1 **W** 1 represents the visit at the end of the 1st week of the 1st four-week OWL Diet cycle (Cycle 1). **C** 2 **W** 4 represents the visit at the end of the 4th week of Cycle 2 (a total of eight weeks on the OWL Diet)

OWL Diet Progress Notes

Name: _____ Starting Date:_____

Starting Weight:_____ Goal Weight:_____ Difference _____

Supplements: B-Complex / Calcium/Vit D / Melatonin / Fiber / K+

HCG: Shots / Cream   125 / 200 / 250

B-12: Med Spa / At Home

Phentermine: _____

Issues: _____

Date: _____ C___ W___

Weight_____   Loss / Gain ____lb(s).   Total Loss _____lb(s).

Hunger: _____

Cheats:_____

Tweaks: _____

BM: _____

Other: _____

Date: _____ C___ W___

Weight _____   Loss / Gain ____ lb(s).   Total Loss _____ lb(s).

Hunger: _____

Cheats: _____

Tweaks: _____

BM: _____

Other: _____

Date: _____ C___ W___

Weight _____   Loss / Gain ____ lb(s).   Total Loss _____ lb(s).

Hunger: _____

Cheats: _____

Tweaks: _____

BM: _____

Other: _____

Date: _____ C___ W___

Weight _____   Loss / Gain ____ lb(s).   Total Loss _____ lb(s).

Hunger: _____

Cheats: _____

Tweaks: _____

BM: _____

Other: _____

PART IV:

GETTING AND STAYING ON TRACK

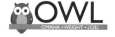

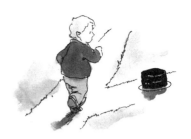

Chapter 15
WHEN PEOPLE
FAIL THE OWL DIET

The OWL Diet does not fail people, but people do fail on the OWL Diet for a variety of reasons.

Weight loss is not easy. You must stay focused and committed to the Low Calorie Diet (LCD).

TIMING IS ESSENTIAL

During initial consultations I do my best to ask people the question: "Is this a good time in your life to commit to losing weight?"

Personal situations that raise a red flag of concern on my part include:

- A recent diagnosis of depression or anxiety
- The start of new psychotropic medications
- A recent life stressor such as starting a new job, a move, loss of a loved one or new health problems
- Recent separation or divorce
- Having just quit smoking
- The need for frequent travel or restaurant dining

On the other hand, one can always argue that you could find an excuse why it is never a good time to lose weight!

People with medical problems that are aggravated by obesity may have been advised that they can no longer delay efforts to lose weight.

For some of us, weight loss is part of reinventing ourselves. Divorce or job loss may help speed the decision to commit to the OWL Diet. Weight loss is often associated with improved self-esteem and enhances existing relationships. Controlling obesity may improve your chances of finding employment or a partner in life.

In every culture, there are events throughout the year that are associated with increased food consumption. It is easy to overeat and gain weight gain during these times. Such events include birthdays, anniversaries, holidays and vacations. These times create potential roadblocks during dieting, and raise the risk of "cheating" (taking in extra food or calories that are not part of the OWL program).

It is important to frankly assess your current life situation to determine if this is the right time for you to commit to the OWL Diet.

When your commitment to success is strong, set a date to begin the diet and focus your activities, thoughts and energy around achieving permanent weight loss.

"I'M STILL HUNGRY"

My experience has been that HCG helps to suppress hunger to varying degrees. At one end of the spectrum, patients come in every week with absolutely no problems with hunger, and I often have to remind them to take in an adequate number of calories to maintain energy and well-being. At the other end of the spectrum are people who come into the med spa every week stating that they are hungry all of the time.

The "I'm still hungry" group is often younger people, typically in their twenties. People in this age group have difficulty following the diet, because much of their social life involves eating out with friends, and consumption of pop or alcoholic beverages. There are many environmental triggers that create food temptations – fast food signs, advertisements on TV and attending live sporting events, to mention just a few.

We have to remember that hunger is cerebral – it starts in your brain, and is affected by emotion. Eating is a behavior to satisfy our urge and food cravings. We no longer eat to survive.

In many cases, our perception of hunger is the real problem.

And let's face it; the LCD requires not only commitment but sacrifice. Uncontrolled feelings of hunger may also be a sign that you are not ready to commit to the LCD. You may have thought you were ready, and you certainly want to succeed, but your life situation may make it especially difficult to adjust to the sacrifices that go with a LCD.

During the initial consultation, and at follow-up appointments, if a patient is complaining of unmanageable hunger, I try to have an honest and open discussion about the timing of participating in the OWL Diet. There may also be some emotional issues that were not fully disclosed at the initial consultation or a critical life situation may have developed. We discuss whether it might be in the best interests of the patient to take a pause in the program and start again at a later date.

In a few patients, the addition of another prescribed appetite suppressant may be appropriate. In the United States, that medication is usually phentermine. A low dose, combined with HCG and the OWL Diet can be very helpful in suppressing appetite. Unlike HCG, phentermine does have the potential for many side effects, including anxiety, insomnia, increased blood pressure and interference with thyroid replacement therapies, so it's not for everyone.

Fortunately, for most of us who have followed the OWL Diet, the use of HCG does help curb our appetite. There will still be days of increased hunger. Hunger may occur on Days Three or Four of the cycle, or even as late as Week Four. We are all different. Part of your commitment to succeed has to be your willingness to work through the hunger.

At times of hunger, try the following:

- Distract your attention by changing activities
- Drink a diet beverage or more water
- Go for a walk
- Call a friend for support
- Eat a breadstick or have one your allowed servings of fruit
- Snack on low calorie dill pickles or celery

When you have your next weekly visit and see an additional weight loss of three to five pounds, you will be glad that you stayed committed!

EXERCISERS

Despite my advice to the contrary, some OWL Diet participants insist on highly active exercising. In my experience, this reverses all of the positive effects of HCG. Exercise that results in a markedly increased heart rate, increased respirations or sweating inevitably drives hunger. Hunger from exercise is hard to ignore and usually results in an increased intake of food, beyond that allowed with my program.

Exercisers will typically arrive in my med spa stating that they are very hungry and "had to eat more calories." When they weigh in, they are even more disappointed to find that they did not lose weight or lost only one to two pounds over the week.

I explain to them once again the need to abstain from high-level exercise. If they listen to my advice, and follow the diet, they are then rewarded the following week with a typical three to five pound weight loss.

If they continue to insist on exercising, they will finish the month feeling miserable, complaining that they were hungry all month, and disappointed with a less than optimal amount of weight loss (if any).

CHEATERS

Cheaters are people who do not follow the OWL Diet protocol. They eat extra calories that are not permitted. The result is no loss of weight or weight loss than is less than optimal.

There may be several reasons for this behavior:

- Low self esteem
- Eating for comfort from emotional stress
- Sleep deprivation causing impaired hunger control
- Self-destructive behavior pattern
- Lack of commitment
- Lack of supportive spouse, friends, family, or co-workers

Some cheaters are honest about consuming extra calories and admit this fact at their weekly visit. This group has the ability to let go of the previous week's failure, understand why they cheated and work to recommit and follow the OWL program as laid out for them.

We all bend the rules sometimes and dieting is no exception. There should be no guilt or shame in having a bad week, as long as one strives to do better. This person earns my respect for being honest, and receives as much support, encouragement and coaching, as he or she needs.

Other cheaters try to hide the fact that they consumed extra calories. This group of people will not do well, as they fail to assume responsibility for their choices. Whatever the cause or excuse for cheating, the reality is that no one force feeds us. It is our brain, hand and mouth that participate in cheating.

If you follow the LCD, you will lose weight. This is simple arithmetic. When your body takes in 600-700 calories in a day, it is looking for an additional source of energy to function and maintain life. With the guidance of HCG, your body chooses fat deposits to draw down, and metabolize for energy. The only exception would be a patient with severe, undiagnosed hypothyroidism. In that scenario, I advise the patient to have his or her thyroid function checked, which is easily done with one test called the Thyroid Stimulating Hormone (TSH). In a severely hypothyroid patient, the TSH will be very high. A borderline result would not explain the inability to lose weight on the LCD.

Ultimately, the dishonest cheater will choose to stop the program. This will be "another diet that did not work." From my point of view, I say that they "fell off the radar" and I usually never hear from them again.

On a positive note, most people do commit to this program, and reap the rewards of rapid and safe weight loss. The result is self-empowering. Each week nearly all the people we see at Omaha Med Spa are the committed ones, who are so very happy with the results that they see. This is a very positive program, with positive outcomes.

TWEAKERS

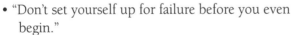

"Tweakers" are people who add certain foods to the OWL Diet, even though they are not recommended or approved. At the initial consultation, when the LCD is reviewed in detail, almost everyone asks to add certain foods to the approved list. This negotiation is met with my uniform responses that range from the following:

- "Don't set yourself up for failure before you even begin."
- "Don't try to reinvent the wheel - the program works as it is set up - don't make changes to it."
- "Put on blinders. Stay focused and stay committed."

"Tweaking" is the very common behavior of adding certain foods, in the hope of having more food variety and taste, and with the hope of still losing weight at the typical rate seen on the OWL Diet.

I want you to succeed. One of the worst behaviors is to "tweak" the diet right out of the starting gates (during the first week) with the outcome of not losing an optimal amount of weight at the end of the first week.

In fact, that was my exact personal experience. I love bananas and stubbornly decided that I should be able to have them as part of my fruit choices. The result was a very slow first week of losing weight. At the start of Week Two, I smartened up and followed my own guidelines with the result that my weight loss kicked into high gear.

Don't "tweak" early on, because there will be times despite your best efforts that you will be forced to "involuntarily tweak." An example would be going out to dinner to celebrate an anniversary. You do your research and choose a restaurant that has its menu posted online. You know ahead of time what you are going to order, but you do not have final control over how that food will be prepared in the kitchen. Suddenly it arrives at the table appearing quite different than what you had expected. You make the best of a challenging moment.

After you have attained at least 50% of your weight loss goal, there are times "approved tweaks" may be attempted - (See Chapter 8). The request to tweak may come out of boredom with the diet. Examples of tweaks that **may** work include: the use of egg whites, tofu, pork tenderloin, turkey and tuna. Add these foods only after consultation with your weight loss doctor and only as a substitution for other approved foods, not as an addition to your daily caloric limits.

SPOUSES, FAMILY, FRIENDS AND CO-WORKERS

Despite their good intentions, your spouse, family, friends and co-workers may be less supportive than you would like, or worse, they may even attempt to sabotage your efforts at weight loss.

The reasons for this are complex. Those who are sabotaging you might not even be aware of what they are doing. Here are a few possible inter-personal dynamics that you may face:

Spouses
- They are more attracted to you as an overweight person
- They feel threatened that you might leave if you lose weight
- They use the low self-esteem that usually accompanies being overweight to their advantage.
- If you lose weight, then they may have to lose weight also
- They like to eat out a lot
- Dieting means not getting together with friends

• They don't support you spending money on "another weight loss program"
• If you lose weight, you will need more clothes, and spend more money

Family and Friends

Many of the spouse sabotage strategies also apply here, but also:

• Worry this is a sign of an eating disorder (especially common in moms)
• Are competitive about who looks best
• Deny that you are actually overweight
• Engage in control and power struggles with you – if you lose weight, you will prove that you are stronger
• Complain that your dieting will ruin family gatherings, especially during holidays

Co-Workers

While many of the above sabotage strategies also apply here, the workplace may be one of the most potentially challenging environments, where some people act in hurtful ways due to:

• Competitiveness for better paying jobs.
• Competitiveness for attention of co-workers, or senior staff.

The workplace is also an area where you cannot control the food that is in the break room. It may be harder to say "no" to a treat when you are at work and everyone else is enjoying a special snack or meal. If a co-worker has brought in a home baked item (perhaps your favorite treat), you may feel a sense of pressure to eat that food, for fear of hurting your co-workers feelings.

THE STEALTH DIET

Due to concerns about how the people around you will react, many OWL Diet participants start out by keeping friends, family, co-workers and even spouses in the dark about what they are doing.

It is very hard to conceal the OWL Diet from your spouse. The first clue would be a dramatic change in your eating habits. Then there is the HCG in the form of shots in the refrigerator or HCG cream in the drawer. They're pretty hard to hide.

I recommend that you have a frank talk with the people in your life who need to know you are on a challenging diet and ask them for their support.

On a positive note, when your spouse, relative, friends and co-workers see how quickly you are losing weight, there is an excellent chance that they will be excited and pleased for you. They may even start the OWL Diet themselves, and join you on the journey to taking control over their own weight problems.

Let me add a final word on buddies. A buddy can be an excellent partner to help you get through the bumps in the road that inevitably come along when you are changing life patterns.

I don't recommend becoming an evangelist for the OWL Diet. That tends to turn people off and turns up the volume of the complaints, cautions and resistance.

Sometimes we choose friends who are of a similar weight, so if your social network or family has several overweight members, you might try asking one or two of them if they would like join you on the OWL Diet. There is strength in numbers!

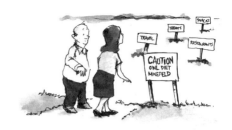

Chapter 16
PROBLEM SOLVING

Even with every possible good intention, you will encounter challenges as you proceed with your OWL Diet. This chapter is intended to help you address those challenges and achieve your weight loss goal.

I'm including a few of the most common issues I have encountered in my personal experience with the OWL Diet that my patients have reported to me.

DINING OUT

The OWL Diet is not conducive to dining out. The best option is to avoid restaurant eating until you achieve your weight loss goal.

This may not be as viable for those who travel as part of their work, or who entertain clients over meals.

With family and friends, it is best to be honest and tell them, "I am on a physician guided diet that prevents me from eating out at this time. Once I am done with this program, I look forward to going out to eat with you." Another option is to change the venue for a meeting. Go out for tea or coffee (without the treats), go to a movie (without the popcorn) or invite friends and family to your home for an evening of board games or musical entertainment.

In your long term maintenance program, it will be important for you to understand that social situations do not always need to include food. When you are feeling strong and committed to your program, venture into the realm of social activities that don't involve food.

A sense of isolation is another pitfall of the OWL Diet, so be aware that, if most of your social activities were around food before the OWL Diet, withdrawal from your social life can be a diet saboteur. Be creative and find new ways to be with friends and family.

TRAVEL

When possible, it is best to participate in the OWL Diet when you do not have any firm travel plans. If work requires you to travel on a regular basis, then you will certainly have some challenges, but with commitment and focus, you can still be successful.

With car travel, always have water in the car and a source of approved foods such as breadsticks, Melba toast, celery, fresh vegetables and fruit.

If you are using injectable HCG, always carry a cooler for your syringes and be sure there is a refrigerator in your hotel room. If you are using HCG cream, make sure the cream is protected from overheating. Avoid leaving HCG cream in the sun, or in an overheated car, since the heat will damage the potency of the HCG.

If you are traveling by air, place your supply of HCG shots with an ice pack and store them in your checked luggage. This works fine if your total travel time is limited to less than four hours

If your travel time is greater, then using the HCG cream with an ice pack would be a safer option. Due to heightened air travel security, the risk of trying to bring the shots or cream in your carry-on luggage is that the airport security may decide to confiscate it from you.

Whether you travel by car or airplane, I strongly advise you to keep a copy of the original prescription for HCG, and a letter from your doctor, explaining why you are traveling with the shots or cream. Despite taking these steps, I have had participants who have their HCG supplies removed from carry-on and checked luggage.

SLEEP AND WEIGHT LOSS

We know that people who do not get enough sleep, or a restful sleep, have trouble with losing weight.

Sleep requirements vary greatly between individuals and may change over the course of your lifetime. Although some people seem to function very well on five hours sleep and others need as much as nine hours sleep per night, the majority of people function very well with an average of seven to eight hours sleep per night.

Unfortunately, in our society, many of us are chronically sleep deprived. There are many causes for this, that are beyond the scope of this chapter. Suffice it to say that this is an important area to address when you're starting the OWL Diet.

Sleep deprivation causes:

- Increased hunger
- Irritability
- Poor decision making (higher risk of "cheating")

Poor quality sleep occurs due to many causes, some of which include:

- Insomnia (difficulty getting to sleep)
- Frequent awakening through the night
- Anxiety and depression
- Snoring
- Sleep apnea
- Bladder or prostate problems
- Family members who have to awaken early to go to work or school
- Excessive use of caffeine or alcohol
- Hormone swings

A significant underlying mood disorder that leads to inadequate sleep must be diagnosed and treated before a person can effectively tackle weight concerns.

Similarly, symptoms such as snoring, awakening with shortness of breath or pauses in breathing at night should be investigated, because they could indicate sleep apnea or heart disease.

The responsibilities of work (sometimes more than one job), raising children, or caring for family members may create challenges that cannot be easily changed or adjusted. Sometimes we have to do the best with the circumstances we are given.

However, there are times that we need to say "no" to those who want us to make new commitments, especially when our energy is focused on the OWL Diet success. There are situations where we have to place our own health and wellness ahead of the call to participate in community or family activities.

CONSTIPATION AND DIARRHEA

If you have a persistent bout of diarrhea on the OWL Diet, then you most likely have an intestinal illness unrelated to dieting. If the symptoms are severe or persistent, you should seek medical attention.

There are some reports of transient diarrhea occurring during the first week of the diet. Other than a viral illness, the possibilities include:

- Excessive fat loading
- Your body adapting to higher (healthier) intake of fresh fruits, salads and vegetables

Even with the healthy allowed intake of water, fruits and vegetables, constipation occurs for many OWL Diet participants. On the LCD, you may find your stool pattern will change. Stool frequency decreases and it is not uncommon to move your bowels every two or three days. If you do not have a bowel movement for more than four days, you should seek medical advice.

An excellent preventative is to use a low-calorie or calorie-free fiber supplement. The addition of stool softeners such as docusate may also be helpful. Check with your doctor to see what option is best for you.

If you are constipated, fiber will not resolve your dilemma, and a laxative is needed. Many effective laxatives are available without a prescription, including the use of either plant-based sennosides (such as Senekot). Another over the counter laxative option is biscacodyl (brand name Dulcolax). Ask your pharmacist or your doctor, and follow the dosing instructions.

Laxatives may cause abdominal pain and cramping – this is normal. If symptoms are severe, or persist, then always seek medical attention, as there can be other reasons for your abdominal pain.

If a first line laxative (Senekot or Dulcolax) does not work, then I suggest the use of liquid magnesium citrate (usually found in drug stores as a generic). I suggest that you chill it well before drinking. Start with a half bottle, or as directed by the pharmacist and label directions. Some patients with reduced kidney function should avoid magnesium citrate altogether. When in doubt, always consult with your doctor.

MUSCLE CRAMPS

Some OWL participants complain of muscle weakness or muscle cramping. This may be the result of the ketoacidosis caused by fat burning, which may cause a drop in potassium levels.

Some patients benefit from the addition of a low dose potassium supplement (often 99 mg. per dose) that is available over the counter. Taken once or twice a day, this may relieve the problem.

You should only take potassium supplements with your doctor's advice since your level of kidney function or certain prescription drugs may also affect potassium levels.

BLURRED VISION

Some people on a LCD report intermittent blurred vision. This may be due to a drop in blood sugar, which can cause changes to the lens of the eye. If the complaint is mild and intermittent, then you can correct it by evenly spacing your calories over the course of your day. If blurred vision is severe or persistent, then seek further medical attention.

LIGHTHEADEDNESS OR DIZZINESS

There are many medical causes of this complaint. It may be a sign of a drop in blood pressure in a patient on blood pressure medication or a drop in blood sugar in a diabetic.

If the symptoms are mild, then check your blood pressure and blood sugar readings. Be sure you are drinking sufficient water. If symptoms are severe, or persistent, see a doctor.

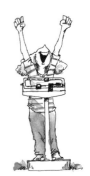

Chapter 17
MAINTENANCE

With the Omaha Weight Loss Diet, you are permitted to go from one cycle (four weeks) directly into the next, until you reach your target weight. This is one key area where the OWL Diet differs from the original Simeons VLCD Diet.

It is safe for you to continue the LCD program for as many months in a row as are needed, due to the higher calorie allowance of the OWL Diet and because we mandate the use of vitamin supplements.

If after two or three months (cycles), you feel you need a break from the program, that is fine. During your break, you must follow the maintenance program.

Whether you have reached your final target weight or you are simply taking a break, your goal is to not gain any weight.

When you are ready to re-start the OWL program, and it has been four weeks or more off of the HCG, then repeat the "fat loading" on Day One and Two of your first resumed cycle. If your maintenance break has been less than four weeks, I advise skipping the fat loading step before restarting the LCD.

Once you achieve your final target weight, you will want to maintain that weight. Most people become very protective of their weight loss.

Unlike the original HCG Protocol from the 1940s, I do not subscribe to using the "phase" terminology. I find it to be obsessive, ritualistic and unnecessary.

Common sense applies during maintenance. You know that you cannot return to the way you ate before, or you will regain your weight.

During the course of the OWL Diet, you have learned:

- You do not need large amounts of oil or grain carbohydrates to have a healthy diet
- Portion control is important

- Eat fresh or frozen foods as much as possible
- Avoid processed foods
- Eat lean meat

In maintenance you may now:

- Go out to eat, but limit portions, avoid sauces and commercial salad dressings and say "no" to desserts except on the rarest of occasions
- Enjoy alcohol, but not more than one or two drinks per day
- Eat limited amounts of fat-free dairy products
- Eat limited amounts of bread and pasta products
- Establish a healthy exercise routine

Your calorie intake in maintenance will vary depending on your age, height and activity level. Follow the guidelines in the box below, or consult with your physician.

Maintenance Calorie Intake:

Here is a simple way to calculate your daily caloric intake once you have reached your goal weight:

Your goal weight in pounds: _____

Your activity level:
  20 = very active men
  15 = moderately active men or very active women
  13 = inactive men or moderately active women and people over age 55
  10 = inactive women

Multiply your goal weight by your activity level: _____

> *Example: a 175-pound moderately active man is 175 x 15 = 2625 calories a day.*

This is your maintenance caloric intake.

To repeat an important point, the key in maintenance is to limit your intake of oil-rich foods and grain carbohydrates.

I do recommend that OWL Dieters wean themselves gradually from HCG by using HCG cream in a maintenance dose of 125 IU on Monday, Wednesday and Friday over ten weeks. After that, no further HCG will be necessary.

My experience has been that unhealthy food cravings do not return unless you go back to the way you ate before the OWL Diet. If you do go back to those old eating patterns of high calorie fats and carbohydrates, your hunger cravings for those foods will return. You will gain your weight back – and then some!

I recently had a patient who had lost 65 pounds on the OWL Diet. She fell off the wagon for just one week, ate lots of fatty foods — and gained 12 pounds! She even admitted she didn't enjoy the fatty foods anymore. Fortunately, she "got it" and realized she was in trouble and came into my office for help. After just a week back on the OWL Diet, she shed those 12 pounds.

EXERCISE

Now is the time to dust off the treadmill, reactivate the gym membership and get some new workout clothes. Now is the time to really step up the exercise. As I said early in this book, exercise is good for you; it just is not a great way to lose weight for most of us.

Exercise is a great way to keep your weight off! Exercise is also proven to reduce your risk for heart disease and high blood pressure. Exercise strengthens bones to reduce the risk of osteoporosis and keeps joints mobile. Working out combats fatigue, enhances sleep and improves mental functioning.

Because you've lost weight - perhaps a great deal of weight - exercise will be easier and more fun. You will find your energy levels are excellent and your enthusiasm for life might even change.

YOUR EATING PLAN

The OWL Diet uses real food instead of processed, manufactured foods. During your weight loss journey, I hope that you have learned to enjoy fresh fruits and vegetables that grow on the earth. If you try processed food just once, I am sure you will discover that the taste is artificial and you will want to avoid these so-called foods that are born in factories.

First, I want to congratulate you for achieving your goal weight. Not only have you improved your health, you have created a lifelong healthy relationship with food that will help you keep the weight off permanently.

Here are some parting tips as you go onto the maintenance phase of the OWL Diet. I like to think you'll stay on it for life:

- Eat real plants, not food that comes from food processing plants.
- Eat your fruits, don't drink them.
- If you can't name the plant or animal that produced the "food," you probably shouldn't eat it.
- Buy your vegetables fresh or frozen. Avoid canned vegetables that have lost much of their nutritional value.
- Start your own garden and enjoy the satisfaction of growing and eating your own food. Community gardens are a great choice for urban dwellers with limited green space. Have a balcony? Start a small container garden. You'll be surprised how much food can grow in a small area!
- Support your local farmers and farmers market.
- Keep reading labels. If you do not recognize the names of the top five ingredients, it's probably not healthy for you. Look at the calories per serving, the number of servings per package, and the number of fat calories. If you do, you may never eat another peanut butter sandwich or frozen pie again.
- Don't grocery shop when you are tired or stressed. You are more likely to make impulsive unhealthy food choices.
- Shop the perimeter of the grocery store. This is where the real food tends to be: fruits, vegetables, meats and dairy. Don't feel compelled to push your grocery cart up and down every aisle.
- Get away from drinking soft drinks altogether.
- Cut back on caffeine or eliminate it altogether.
- Plan your meals for the week. The OWL Diet has taught you to organize and always have healthy food choices on hand.
- Prepare meals in advance and always take food to work.
- If you choose to eat dairy products (most of us do), go back to enjoying them in low-fat or fat-free forms, such as: skim milk, almond milk, fat-free yogurt, low fat cheese – mozzarella, fresh goat, feta, grated Parmesan and 1% cottage cheese.
- Start enjoying breakfast again! Choose healthy cereals that contain whole grains, oats and are low in sugar. Treat yourself to the oc-

casional poached egg. Buy breads that are rich in whole grains, and limit yourself to 1 slice per day.

- You are now allowed to enjoy rice, potatoes and pasta again! Hurray! Go slow and keep those portion sizes small.
- Stay away from deep-fried anything.
- Enjoy salmon again.
- Re-start those fish oil capsules that you used to take.
- Limit your intake of fish that are at the top of their food chain, such as tuna and swordfish, due to the risk of mercury contamination.
- In America we tend to eat like we are in a huge hurry. Slow down – taste the food you eat – savor the flavors. Stop eating before you are completely full.
- Don't do anything else when you are eating—no television or reading. A pleasant conversation with your family is fine.
- Dine out occasionally, but learn to say "no" to the bread that comes before the salad, not to speak of the dessert cart.
- Consider an appetizer as your complete meal, or order an entrée and have the server place half of it in a take home container before it even arrives at your table.
- Treats are just that – treats. They are not meant to be a part of your daily eating habit. Enjoy a dessert – but limit yourself to once per week.
- If you want ice cream, buy it in a small single serving from the grocery store. Pails are meant for sand castles, not for take home ice cream.
- Try frozen yoghurt or sorbets instead of fat-laden regular ice cream.
- If you want a cookie – buy a cookie, not a bag of them.
- Want a piece of pie? That's fine, but buy it by the piece and not the whole pie.
- Don't eat supper at the cinema. You should be going for the movie, not the popcorn.
- No more supersizing of anything! I encourage you to avoid all forms of junk food - made from potatoes, corn or other grains – or anything that looks like some form of chip. The oil content is simply too high. By reading the calorie content on a bag of potato chips I'm sure you will agree.
- Become aware of the corn content in the food that you eat. The majority of our manufactured foods now come from corn, and there

is a growing awareness that this may be part of the problem of the "Western Diet" that is so prone to causing cancer, heart disease and diabetes.

- Avoid high fructose corn syrup (a corn by-product) that has permeated our food supply.

- Enjoy a full range of meats, including lean pork and turkey. Learn from the OWL Diet that you should always avoid eating the skin from fowl like chicken and turkey.

- Olive oil is the preferred oil for cooking, when it is called for. Remember that 1 tablespoon of olive oil is approximately 120 calories! A small bottle should last a very long time.

- Continue to enjoy fresh limes and lemons in your diet. Make Braggs Liquid Aminos your ongoing choice for soy sauce. Explore some of the other low-calorie/fat-free dressings that are now available and you may now use to flavor your salads.

- Consider eating from smaller plates at home. The size of our dinner plate has actually increased over the past few decades, making us think we need to fill it up.

- Leave serving bowls in the cupboard. Dish up your food directly to your plate in the correct serving size. When you are finished, do not go back for seconds. Learn to love leftovers!

- When you were on the OWL Diet, I encouraged you not to weigh yourself every day, but rather weekly at your doctor's office. Now I want you to weigh at home every day! If your weight goes up by more than three pounds, then you need to start cutting calories again until it gets back to normal.

- Go see your regular doctor, if you have not been in for a while. Show off your new weight and feel the sense of accomplishment that you deserve.

I am proud of you for taking control over your weight. Well done! You did it the natural way – with real food. And you have learned how to eat better. You can now go on and lead a healthier life.

You look better in the mirror, better in pictures and better in the new clothes! Your confidence and self-esteem are at all-time highs! Congratulations!

Stay up to date with future enhancements to the Omaha Weight Loss Diet by following Dr. Carter Abbott at: www.OWLDiet.com.

About the Author

Carter Abbott received his Doctor of Medicine degree from the University of Western Ontario in London, Ontaro, Canada in 1983. He has been a primary care physician in both Canada and the United States. His interests have taken him to both urban and rural settings, clinics and hospitals, nursing homes and palliative care facilities, urgent care clinics and emergency room care. This diverse practice experience of over 25 years has equipped him with a unique understanding of the obesity problem that faces many of us. During his personal journey to successful permanent weight loss, he developed the Omaha Weight Loss Diet – OWL Diet for short. The OWL Diet is the basis for this book. Stay up to date on the Owl Diet by visiting Dr. Abbott's website: www.OWLDiet.com.

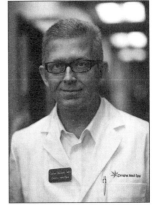

Dr. Carter O. Abbott, M.D.